TINA VINDUM'S
OUTDOOR
FITNESS

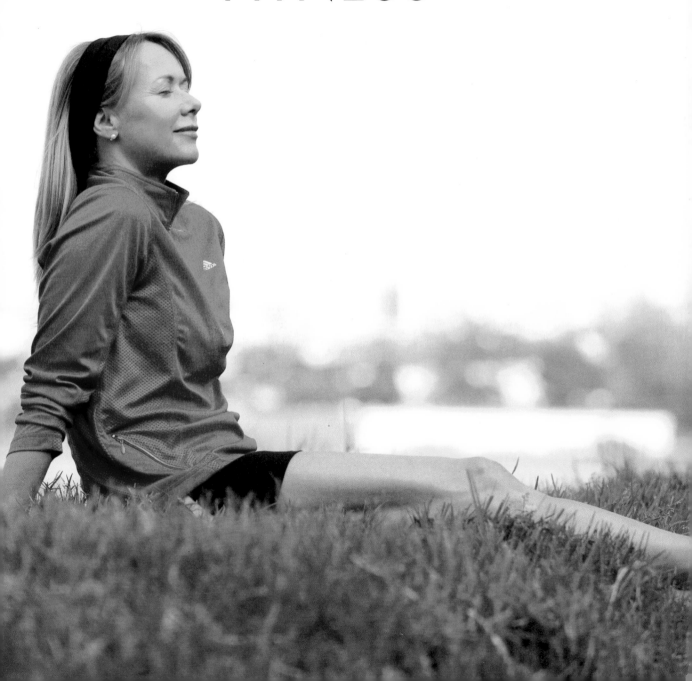

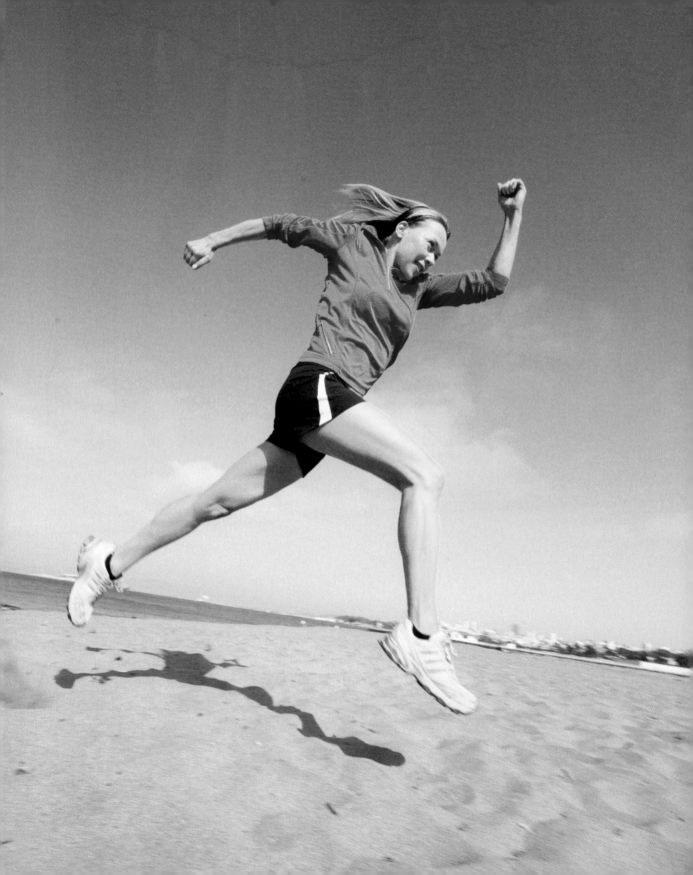

TINA VINDUM'S
OUTDOOR
FITNESS

Step Out of the Gym and Into the BEST Shape of Your Life

The Revolutionary Approach to True
BodyMind Fitness in as Little as 8 Weeks

Tina Vindum

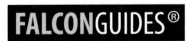

GUILFORD, CONNECTICUT
HELENA, MONTANA

An imprint of The Globe Pequot Press

For John, with whom life is one continuous BodyMind adventure.

To buy books in quantity for corporate use
or incentives, call **(800) 962–0973**
or e-mail **premiums@GlobePequot.com**.

Falcon, FalconGuides, and Outfit Your Mind are registered trademarks of Morris Book Publishing, LLC.

Interior photos © Adam Brown Photography, except as noted; chapter opener photos © Shutterstock
Project manager: Julie Marsh
Layout artists: Melissa Evarts, Casey Shain
Text design by Sheryl P. Kober
Library of Congress Cataloging-in-Publication Data is available on file.
ISBN 978-0-7627-5129-7

Printed in the United States of America
10 9 8 7 6 5 4 3 2 1

Medical Disclaimer

Starting a new fitness regimen should begin with making a candid assessment of your current health and fitness level. Under certain circumstances you should seek a doctor's approval before you begin the Outdoor Fitness program. If you have any questions about your health, you should consult your physician before beginning this or any fitness program.

CONTENTS

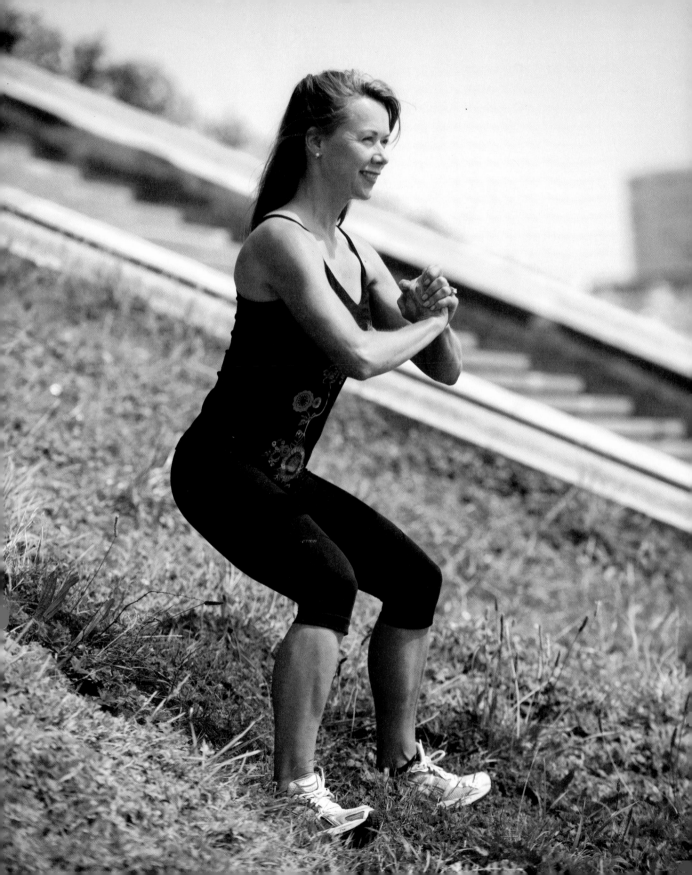

INTRODUCTION

I remember distinctly the moment that my approach to fitness was transformed. As both a former Alpine skier and competitive mountain biker, I had spent years of my life in a gym. Training and keeping fit was my job. Over time, I had been growing increasingly frustrated with training in the static indoor environment: those workout rooms full of stationary bikes and treadmills, weight machines, and fluorescent lights. Working out day after day, I could feel my mind and body going numb in this dull, oxygen-deprived, monochromatic environment. It was also getting harder and harder to really test and challenge my body. My muscles had grown so used to the repetitive exercises of standard gym equipment, I had reached a plateau that was taking away from my performance.

One day I found myself staring out the window in the middle of yet another boring indoor workout, gazing at the majestic Sierra Nevadas, feeling stifled and frustrated. It was fall, training season for skiing. Leaves covered the ground, and the air was crisp and cold. Like a kid stuck in a classroom, I pined for the freedom that lay outside my window. That day, I rebelled. I threw on extra layers of clothes and took my workout outside. Soon I was running slalom through the pine trees, learning to keep my balance on the uneven terrain, and stopping from time to time to do strengthening and stretching exercises against the tree trunks and boulders. Using the diverse terrain of the Sierras, that day I created an alternative gym with a thousand possibilities and an exciting new way to exercise and train my body. It was a thrilling experience to use the natural surroundings to guide my workouts and to discover that I didn't need a lot of equipment to achieve muscular strength, agility, and power. I knew instantly that this was the workout I'd been longing for: an intuitive, brand-new way to exercise and improve my performance; a way to keep my training continually fresh and challenging; a way to feed my mind and spirit as well as work my body.

That afternoon in the Sierras, I started to create the program you're about to begin, Outdoor Fitness, a holistic approach to fitness that honors the interconnection of body, mind, emotion, and the environment.

After spending some time training in the outdoors, I began to notice some unexpected changes: a noticeable increase in my mental focus and sharpness, a sense of emotional strength, and greater well-being that infused me with a post-workout calm and centeredness I had never quite achieved before. I was getting great physical results, and I was also getting a whole lot more. I began to experience happiness and joy—it was as if every cell in my body was overflowing with a new life force. I had reconnected with that place inside me that loved being outside and near nature, that place where I was a "kid" again, a place that now I cannot live without.

Very quickly, this new approach to training showed up in my results. I was winning races, achieving new personal records, and reaching a new level of performance on the mountain—and in my life. Skiing nonstop runs down Heavenly's famed Gunbarrel run drew the attention of one of the most published outdoor sports photographers at the time, Larry Prosor. This photo shoot also led to others with world-class pho-tographers, including Bruce Weber, Lori Adamski-Peek, Scott Markewitz, and John Kelly. I became a sponsored athlete for companies including Fila, Salomon, Oakley, Roces, Fisher, Hind, and Scott. I even won a World Championship medal in mountain biking.

Soon everyone wanted to know what I'd been doing to get in such great shape. I began to share my new approach and techniques with fellow skiers, as well as other athletes, who experienced the same joy and excitement that I'd felt that first day on the trail. They also achieved the same results: They became stronger, faster, and more flexible; sharpened their mental focus and felt more centered and calm; and discovered a new competitive edge. Most profoundly, they felt renewed passion for exercise and a new connection to the natural world.

A few short years later, I became a professional fitness trainer and combined my certified expertise with my passion for the outdoors into a trademarked Outdoor Fitness program—the only outdoor exercise course to be accredited by the fitness field's two leading professional institutions, the American Council on Exercise (ACE) and the Aerobics and Fitness Association of America (AFAA).

Outdoor Fitness, which can be tailored to athletes, trainers, and women and men of all ages, backgrounds, and fitness levels, has gained a national and international following. As a personal trainer recently said after attending one of my workshops, "I was so inspired and lifted in so many ways from the information and the experience . . . my brain was on fire as I drove back home . . . I know without a doubt I too can fulfill and deliver to my community an incredible workout outdoors that gets results along with the awesome feeling of doing it outdoors."

I've spent more than a decade honing Outdoor Fitness, taking it from a workout plan I used to help fellow professional skiers train more effectively to a certified and world-renowned program used to train hundreds of personal trainers, coaches, and athletes around the globe. In pursuit of true whole health, it combines physical fitness techniques with cutting-edge information on fitness physiology, nutrition, mental health, and wellness.

Outdoor Fitness is based on a combination of my unique set of exercises: Base Moves and Signature Moves, which are exercises that can be done in any outdoor location or site, including hilly or mountainous trails, a city or suburban park, a beach or a rural setting. By utilizing a variety of terrain, you will learn a new degree of body awareness and train your body to move in a variety of ways. Rather than moving in a linear direction, as on a treadmill or stair-stepper, you will soon be moving forward, backward, diagonally, laterally, and up and down. Using a variety of movement patterns over different types of terrain taxes the body in all planes of movement, increases the stability of your muscles and joints, and burns more fat and calories.

Outdoor Fitness is built around three basic types of workouts: single site, multisite, and traveling. Single-site workouts are one-spot sessions, which you can do in parks, in playgrounds, or right in your own backyard. Multisite workouts allow you to incorporate at least two different terrains or locations during a session, such as two or more stops along a stretch of beach or hillside. Traveling workouts are just what they sound like: sessions where the workout literally travels from one place to another throughout the allotted time, such as a 1- to 5-mile loop up to a mountain meadow and back down through the woods.

Outdoor Fitness has three phases, each comprising four weeks. Each phase ensures clear, measurable results in all aspects of the workout—physical skills and changes, mental focus and clarity, and emotional calm and well-being—but also offers you a clear road map to lose weight, increase your lean muscle mass, increase your cardiovascular health, and achieve a slender but stronger physique. The design of Outdoor Fitness is based on my belief that for an exercise program to truly work and stick with you, it needs not only to incorporate strength, endurance, agility, balance, flexibility, and kinesthetic awareness, but also the tools to develop mental focus and emotional power. The extraordinary gift is the use of environmental integration techniques that pull the BodyMind fitness together.

Each phase builds on the phase that comes before and becomes increasingly challenging. If you're an experienced athlete, you might be tempted to skip Phase 1, looking for a tougher workout. Don't do it. Taking the time to get to know my Base Moves and Signature Moves, as well as my approach to fitness in general, will help you grasp the program and avoid injury. You'll also maximize your physical, mental, and emotional results by starting at the beginning. Each phase is full of adaptations to increase or decrease the degree of challenge, so that whether you feel you are a beginner, intermediate, or advanced, you will be able to meet your workout needs and your desired degree of difficulty. Throughout the three phases, you will find supportive and encouraging tips on how to keep track of your progress,

manage your goals, and recover from breaks in your routine.

The goal of Phase 1: Building Your Base is to become familiar with my approach to fitness, learn proper alignment and positioning for the Base Moves, and get comfortable exercising outdoors. You will learn specific techniques, including how to "feel through your feet"; how to breathe in a way that creates more energy and enhances the intimate relationship between you, your body, and the environment; and how to develop posture that enhances your mood. During this phase you will rewire your brain, creating new, positive thought patterns for and about exercise. You'll learn how to improve your mental focus and acuity with several techniques that tap into your own emotional power. You'll also learn a new way to view and utilize the outdoors—whether your environment is your own backyard, an urban park, a suburban neighborhood, a field or a meadow in a rural setting, the beach, the mountains, or the woods. Perhaps the best feature of Phase 1 is the experience of bringing pure, simple fun back into your exercise routine. Remember the feeling of being a kid playing outdoors—the freedom of movement, the endless curiosity, the dirt and sweat you accumulated like a badge of honor at the end of a long afternoon of rambling around? That's what I call "clean dirty fun," and it's what Outdoor Fitness is all about. Forget boredom. It simply doesn't exist with this program.

In Phase 2: Core of Your Core, you build on the physical skills, strength, and mindset that you've established in Phase 1 and ramp it up. By expanding the variety of terrain, integrating more multidirectional movements, and including compound and combo moves, you will go from feeling pretty good to really good. During this phase, you will be able to target and measure your body composition results (a program that I developed in partnership with Dr. Adrian Rawlinson and the California Pacific Orthopedic and Sports Medicine study) and become much more athletic. Since weight loss is a huge topic that is often misleading, I call it body composition. Knowing your muscle-to-fat ratio is all-encompassing: lose fat, gain and maintain muscle. Physically you will learn how to increase your strength, endurance, agility, balance, flexibility, and kinesthetic and proprioceptive awareness. You will also learn more BodyMind techniques, including what I call HeartBrain, PMJ, and Thanksuary. The movements in Phase 2 become a bit more challenging, but they are even more invigorating!

In Phase 3: Sustenance, Outdoor Fitness has become a part of your life. You rev up the duration and intensity of the exercises and perform at a higher level. Although Phase 3 is designed to achieve results in four weeks, like all the phases, this phase is truly all about sustaining your level of health and fitness for the rest of your life. You'll have the skills and experience to keep creating new workouts, new goals, and new challenges for years to come. The best part is you'll actually want to exercise. The way you'll feel, and the benefits you'll see in your body, will make you look forward to getting outside for your sessions.

Learning the basics of Outdoor Fitness is only the beginning of your new fitness adventure. My program opens up a world of workout options that mean you'll never again have to repeat the same tired routine inside your gym. Once you learn the Base and Signature Moves and understand how to scout a workout site, you can either follow my designed workouts or create your own, designing your own combination of moves and adapting sessions to your specific environment and particular goals. In a single week, you might do a single-site workout in a suburban park area for 30 to 60 minutes, followed by a multisite workout that moves you from a flat grassy field up a wooded hillside, capped off by a traveling workout along a peaceful river path. Along the way, you test your body and mind's ability to adapt and adjust to the changing terrain and environmental circumstances. You awaken your brain as you strengthen your body's balance, agility, and core muscle strength. You constantly challenge yourself physically, mentally, and emotionally, in new ways every day, with every session.

The ancient Greeks—creators of the Olympics, a pinnacle of physical skill and mental dedication—were devoted to the quest to live at the highest human potential, physically, mentally, and spiritually. This was *Areté*, defined as an honorable course of thought, feeling, and action; goodness, excellence, and virtue. An individual who possessed *Areté* lived a life shaped around the quest for one's deepest well-being and highest purpose, striving to realize one's full potential in all realms of sport and life. This is my wish for you: a life of *Areté*. Outdoor Fitness is my way to help you achieve it.

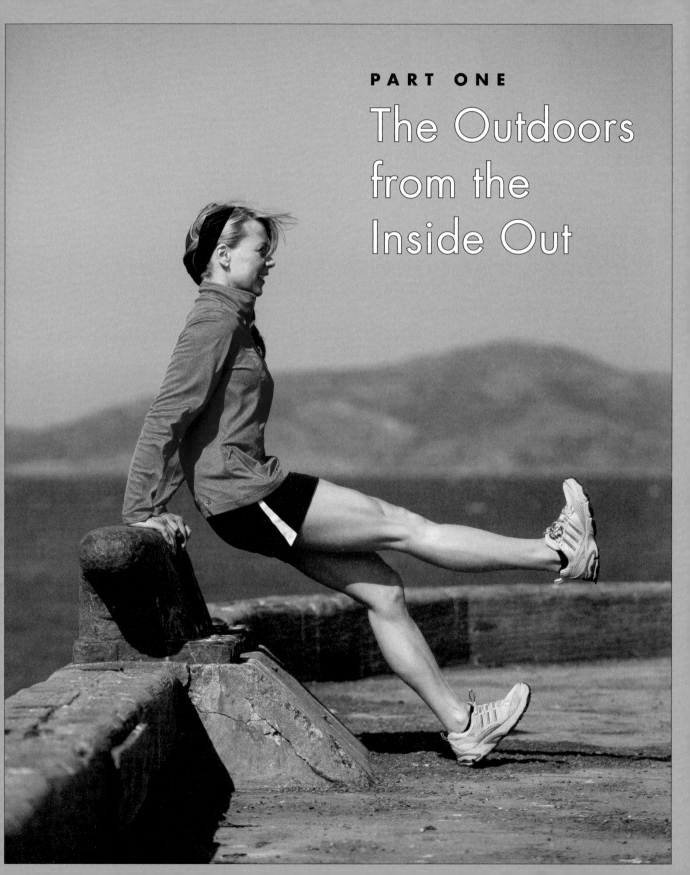

PART ONE

The Outdoors from the Inside Out

CHAPTER 1

The Power of Outdoor Fitness

Imagine you are stepping lightly over grass and fallen leaves, your feet sinking into the softness underfoot. You feel your body warming as your feet, legs, and arms begin to move and find their rhythm. You notice the grass and leaves are still a bit wet from the dew—or did it rain last night? You don't mind. You feel the sun warming your face. You breathe, taking in the slightly musty smell of the molten leaves. You listen to the early-morning birds calling to one another. You hear cars passing in the distance outside the park. Thoughts of the coming day enter your mind—you let them pass. You breathe in, you breathe out, savoring each moment. Your skin begins to tingle and then break a light sweat as your pace increases. Your body feels alive with adrenalin, endorphins, and energy.

Feeling through your feet, the ground seems to be talking to you. You feel the muscles down the entire length of your legs flex and release as you move. Your abs are firm; your back feels strong and supple. The tightness in your hips and aches in your knees have melted away. It's the start of a new day, a new day to move your body, awaken your mind, and renew and revitalize your spirit. You've never felt clearer, stronger, and more comfortable in your own skin.

This is Outdoor Fitness, the most advanced method available today to achieve true BodyMind power and the highest degree of overall fitness, health, and well-being. Over the next 12 weeks, you will transform your body and your whole approach to exercise. You'll gain muscle strength and cardiovascular power, increase your flexibility and endurance, and sharpen your mental skills and emotional health—and you'll do it all outdoors, immersed in the beauty, peace, and tranquility of nature. While you're getting fit like you've never been before, you will also be renewing a powerful personal connection to the natural world, one that will feed not just your body but also your soul.

Maximize Your Results

Here's the first, most important thing to know: Whatever fitness results you can achieve inside the gym, you can—and will—quadruple in the outdoors. This is true whether you live at the base of a mountain, on a crowded city block, or on a suburban cul-de-sac. In Outdoor Fitness, you will use all aspects of your surroundings—from mountain trails to urban city parks, from hillsides to playground benches, from trees to parking meters—to create workouts that are more challenging, and more fun, than anything you've done in the gym. The natural world right outside our doors is actually the most superior gym imaginable—for our bodies, our souls, and ultimately, our consciences! (After all, what is exercising outdoors if not *literally* going green?)

You've made the decision to seek a new fitness regimen, for any number of reasons. Maybe you want to lose weight. Maybe you're looking to improve your cardiovascular health. Maybe you'd like to reduce the stress in your life or help to alleviate the symptoms of illness, such as diabetes, depression, or Seasonal Affective Disorder (SAD). Maybe you're an athlete already, looking to improve your sports performance. Maybe you'd like to reduce your carbon footprint—treadmills, after all, use shocking amounts of energy. Maybe you're simply looking for some much-needed motivation. No matter what brings you to Outdoor Fitness, everyone has one fundamental desire in common: We all want to feel inspired again!

The Outdoor Fitness program is based on my core belief that nature is a powerful—if not the most powerful—contributor to personal health and fitness. When you work out in the fresh air, you not only enhance your physical, mental, and emotional condition, you also deepen the connection you have with yourself, others, and the environment. You'll discover that while exercising in the outdoors brings you to new levels of health, it also brings constant inspiration.

Outdoor Fitness isn't only about inspiration, however; it's also about results. This 12-week program:

- Changes body composition, so that you lose fat, increase muscle, and become leaner and lighter

- Enhances cognitive function, increasing mental focus and performance
- Increases energy level, balances hormones and neurotransmitters, and enables greater emotional equilibrium
- Significantly increases self-confidence, positive body image, and motivation level
- Strengthens the immune system, reduces healing time, and boosts stress response
- Improves the cardiovascular system, shores up bone health, and can reverse type 2 diabetes

Just like you can become addicted to the high a drug can give, your body—and mind—can get hooked on how full of energy, happiness, and even joy you experience doing my program. My client Shelly described it this way: "Wow—the Outdoor Fitness program really changed my life. I could write a book about it." Her experience was so transformative that she detailed the exact ways in which her life changed for the better. This is her list of ways in which she was transformed, straight from her journal!

What others see:
- Less of me! I've lost 10 pounds and reduced my body mass by two dress sizes.
- More energy, greater sense of well-being, noticeably more confidence.
- People often tell me, "You look so athletic and healthy"—a first for me!
- Upbeat attitude—a together person, maybe even a little sexy!

What I see:
- A more feminine, less self-conscious woman—I am comfortable in my skin for the first time in my life.
- I don't see a perfect body, but I'm proud of my forty-year-old self, and I often feel sexy.
- I used to feel like an imposter in hip-hugging, fitted clothes, and now I feel like I belong in them—that's a huge victory for me.

How I feel:
- Personally powerful and balanced.
- Strong, smart, and beautiful.
- Grateful and aware of the beauty of the earth, the nature we have in our backyard, and the inspiration of others in the program.
- I've learned that "someday" is life deferred. I now have the love, energy, and focus to pursue my dreams—now, not later.

Like so many of my clients, Shelly experienced a complete transformation of her life—from the inside out. This capacity for greater contentment—even joy—can be yours as well. Simply put, along with the terrific physical results that come with outdoor exercise, the larger payoff is the feeling of well-being that this program gives you.

The Power of Nature

Why is it so important for us to connect with nature and be outdoors? Because mounting research shows the profound effect that fresh air, plants, trees, and natural outdoor elements have on our health and well-being. When you spend time outdoors, especially being active, you can lift your mood, think more positively, feel more internal calm, and experience greater harmony with the world around you.

Recent studies have shown that being in a natural, outdoor environment is one of the very best things you can do for your health. The findings include:

• Levels of serotonin, a neurotransmitter that helps regulate our mood, rise when we are outside. A study conducted at the University of Queensland in Australia found that regular outdoor runners were less anxious and depressed than people who ran indoors on a treadmill, and they had higher levels of post-exercise endorphins, the feel-good brain chemicals associated with "runner's high."

• Exposure to nature reduces pain and illness and speeds recovery time. In one study of postoperative patients, those who had rooms with a view of natural surroundings needed less pain medication and spent fewer days in the hospital than those who faced a brick wall. In another study, prisoners in Michigan who were able to view sky, grass, and trees had 24 percent fewer infirmary visits and significantly fewer digestive illnesses and headaches.

• Being in nature reduces stress-related anger and enhances sociability. Frances Kuo, a researcher at the University of Illinois, has shown that being around grass and greenery reduces rates of domestic violence and school truancy and leads to better grades and increased social interaction. And a study by Dr. David Lewis, the man who coined the term road rage, found that the scent of grass has a significant calming effect on out-of-control drivers.

• You do your lungs a favor when you exercise outdoors: According to the Environmental Protection Agency (EPA), indoor air in the United States is two to five times more polluted than outdoor air (meaning the outdoor air is 75 percent less polluted than indoor air!). Fresh air is also rich in negative ions (oxygen molecules with an extra electron). These negative ions have been linked to an improved sense of well-being, heightened awareness and alertness, decreased anxiety, and a lower resting heart rate.

Outdoor Fitness not only delivers all of these very real physiological benefits, it also offers you an easy-to-follow, scientifically based, exhilarating way to exercise outdoors. Whether you are looking to begin a new exercise program, you're bored and frustrated with the one you have, or you are looking to increase your sports performance, you will discover a new sense of vitality, confidence, and sheer pleasure of being alive—as you get in the best shape of your life. We don't all need to pick up stakes and move to the woods or the mountains in order to reestablish our health, but we do need to spend time outside. The EPA estimates that we spend more than 90 percent (many scientists argue this number is higher) of our time indoors, inside our homes, our offices, and our cars—we rarely connect with nature and the outdoors.

Feeding on Sunlight

It's easy to forget when we spend too much time indoors, but we need sunlight for our basic well-being. The amount of natural light we take in has an effect on our mood and our physical health. Sunlight directly affects the levels of serotonin and the hormone melatonin created in our bodies. When we have sufficient serotonin levels, we feel suffused with a sense of well-being—we feel calm, alert, capable. Lack of sunlight—and the lack of serotonin that comes with it—is linked to Seasonal Affective Disorder, PMS, depression, irritability, weight gain, alcohol abuse, and migraines. Our sleep is disrupted when we don't generate enough melatonin, which is released in darkness and helps regulate our biological clock, aiding us to sleep.

How Much Sunlight Do You Need?

For most people a minimum of 20 minutes per day of sunlight is necessary for hormonal regularity. People who suffer from Seasonal Affective Disorder may need as much as two hours per day to maintain hormonal stability.

The Limits of the Gym

It's a scientific fact: Our bodies are smart. They look for the easy route, the path that requires the least amount of work. This means our bodies adapt quickly to exercise patterns. So in a gym workout, whether you're using equipment, free weights, or a circuit training machine, your body will quickly learn what it has to do and will switch on autopilot, exerting the least amount of effort possible to complete the task. This is why you reach a plateau so quickly and why the results you get in a gym setting eventually taper off. It's nearly impossible to reach your full potential exercising this way.

In the outdoors, your body is con-

Michelle, Age 30

During her initial consultation, Michelle ran down the list of exercises she performed during an average week. She'd been working with a personal trainer three days per week, riding her mountain bike two days per week, and performing yoga to "destress" one day per week. She'd been on this schedule for two years. When asked about her goals, she said she'd like to lose 20 pounds and gain stamina. Asked how long she'd had these goals, she flatly replied, "Two years."

Wait a minute! What's the problem here? Simply put, Michelle's program had become stale. It was time to disconnect the autopilot, wake up her body and mind, and break through to a whole new level of fitness—mentally and physically.

Michelle began training with Outdoor Fitness the following week and was introduced to a whole new way of looking at health and fitness. She learned about taking a training program and turning it into a lifestyle—and did she ever! She left the interior design profession, learned about fitness, got certified as a personal trainer, and then became certified as an Outdoor Fitness trainer.

It took Michelle just three months to achieve her goal. "I was never able to achieve this with my personal trainer," she said. "I have lost 8 percent body fat, gained strength and mental clarity, increased my productivity at work, I'm more patient with my son, and I feel more centered than I've ever been in my life. I've even stopped seeing my therapist!"

Darlene Quigg, Age 70

Darlene began working out with me when she had just retired from teaching kindergarten and second grade. "Grumpy and disenchanted with how my friends were going gray and getting heavy, I happened upon an article in the local paper about Tina and Outdoor Fitness, and I said, 'Wow!'" So began a five-year stretch that continues today. "Over a period of weeks, I could feel my cardio and legs get stronger. I had more energy. I was sleeping well at night, and I was feeling so much better—it was amazing. At the time, one of my children was going through a crisis, and I found I had so much more patience and calmness to deal with the situation. I keep saying to myself, 'I'm 70'—I just can't believe how good I feel!"

stantly adapting to new actions as it moves up, down, diagonally, or side to side. You are constantly recruiting new muscle fiber, which in turn sends your neurons and muscles new information all the time. This keeps your brain active and engaged. It also keeps your body continually challenged, becoming stronger, faster, and more agile. You'll hear me say over and over again: Life is not a linear event! We as human beings are built for variety and challenges—both mental and physical—that the gym simply can't accommodate.

What's more, indoor gyms are a breeding ground for germs. There are plenty of warm, moist areas that are perfect for generating all kinds of germs, from viruses and bacteria to fungi. Recently, the so-called superbug MRSA

has been spreading to health clubs, causing antibiotic-resistant staph infections. That's due to the fact that while working out, people often sweat, cough, or sneeze, leaving behind germs that can spread the common cold, influenza, skin infections, and many other types of disease.

Then there's the boredom factor. Admit it: No matter how much you care about your health and fitness, you get tired of the same old routine at the gym. It's no surprise since you're not getting much mental stimulation from pumping muscles and heart rates on indoor weight machines, treadmills, and stationary bikes. Most gyms across the country have a staggering 90 percent dropout rate. In contrast, over its history the Outdoor Fitness program has had a

20 percent dropout rate. This is a workout program you'll want to stick with—for its results, and for the great variety that keeps you from ever feeling stifled or bored.

Traditional gym workouts limit your physical progress, expose you to germs and disease, and dampen your motivation with their stale environments and their repetitive, unchanging sessions. It's high time for a change, and here's how it works.

Clean Dirty Fun

I like to call my workouts "clean dirty fun" because each and every workout appeals to our sense of play and adventure. Childhood is the stage when people typically spend the greatest amount of time outdoors at play—running, jumping, and skipping. We can experience that same fun as adults in Outdoor Fitness. Leaping across streams, hopping from rock to rock on a trail, or dashing through a playground—the training's mix of grit, sweat, and fun is youth enhancing. You'll love how your fitness level increases, and you'll also love the deep sense of accomplishment that comes from having braved the terrain and conditions of the outdoors. As Darlene, age 70, said, "I feel so alive in this workout. The smells and the birds. You look up at the redwood trees on the trail, and it's magnificent. When I'm out there breathing the fresh air, all my stress is removed. It's a tremendous cleansing process."

Energy Is at the Core of Health and Fitness

At the most basic level, exercise is all about energy. Energy is the key to life. Without it, our cells cannot function, our

Circulation: Your Lymphatic System

Deep breathing has a powerful effect on your body's lymphatic system, a major component of your immune system. Made up of lymph nodes, ducts, vessels, and organs, your lymph system is a kind of cleaning system for your body, transporting waste and cellular by-products. The lymphatic system has no pump, like your heart, to circulate its fluid. Deep breathing has been shown to stimulate the lymphatic system and increase the rate of toxic elimination by as much as 15 to 20 times the body's normal pace.

bodies cannot move, our brains cannot think. Lack of energy is the first step toward illness and disease. In our bodies, energy originates in our cells. Cells and their mitochondria are the power plants—the energy producers—in your body, providing you with the fuel you need to live healthfully. The oxygen we take in during exercise not only burns fat, it also fuels these energy-producing cells.

It All Begins with *Breath*

Proper breathing is essential for increasing and maintaining energy. It's also the moment-to-moment, day-to-day pathway to whole health. Your breath feeds your brain with cell-powering oxygen and fuels your body's circulation. Breathing deeply cleanses the internal system, and it supports mental clarity and emotional balance. Blood pressure can drop, and stress and anxiety can diminish, when you breathe fully and deeply. When

you're feeling fatigued and stressed out, the first thing you should check is your breathing.

Your breath is also one of the most basic connections to your environment. Every time you breathe in and out, you receive from and give back to your natural surroundings. It's a simple, profound connection—and learning to breathe well will enhance it.

What's the difference between breathing well and breathing poorly? It all starts with the diaphragm, the primary muscle in breathing, located at the boundary between the chest cavity and the abdominal cavity. When you breathe properly, your diaphragm contracts and your abdomen protrudes; this allows your lungs to fill with air. Inside your lungs is where oxygen truly enters your body, through 300 million aveoli, most densely located in the lungs' lower lobes. Thoracic breathing, which is often shallow and gasping, does not engage the diaphragm and prevents your lungs from taking in the maximum

Low and Slow

Many times during your workouts, I'll remind you to breathe low and slow. Breathing low and slow means breathing deeply—into the lower lobes of your lungs for greater oxygenation. It also means keeping control of your breath, not gasping or racing through breaths.

Breathing from Your Diaphragm—An Exercise

Take a breath in. Exhale slowly and completely out of your mouth, releasing air until there is nothing left to exhale. Repeat: breathe in and slowly breathe out, observing how your body works to breathe. What can you observe about your breath?

You probably noticed that when you exhale completely, your body automatically takes in more air. Your lungs work like a vacuum, expanding to draw in the maximum amount of air. Often we think of an exhale as the conclusion of breath, when in fact exhaling is the first step in preparing your body to receive a full, oxygen-rich, diaphragmatic breath.

amount of oxygen. This shallow breathing can cause tension, stress, and anxiety, as well as dizziness and high blood pressure. In a workout, thoracic breathing causes shortness of breath, cramps, muscle pain, tension, fatigue, weakness, and loss of concentration.

The Biophilia Effect

The Outdoor Fitness program is based on my core belief that nature is perhaps the most powerful source for personal health and fitness. When you work out in the fresh air, you not only enhance your physical-mental-emotional condition, you also deepen the connection you have with the environment. It's easy to overlook, since most of us spend so much time indoors, but you and I, like all human beings, have a deep connection to the natural world. Instinctively you know this to be true. This connection to nature is what is called the "biophilia effect."

The concept of *biophilia*, which literally means "love of life," was first hypothesized by Harvard biologist E.O. Wilson. Wilson theorized that human beings have an intrinsic and emotional affiliation to other living things. Simply, we are drawn to other life. This is a deep, genetic affinity rooted in our DNA, the vestige of what was, for early humans, a key to survival. The bond we carry inside us to nature's many forms of life is that primal and that powerful.

For a personal glimpse into biophilia, think about your very own home. Do you keep plants in your living room, flowers in window boxes, or tend a garden? Do you have pets: a cat curled up on your couch, a dog bounding around in the backyard, a goldfish swimming around in a fish tank? Do you light candles or stoke a fire in your fireplace, and do you feel soothed when surrounded by the soft light of flame? These are all examples of ways we bring nature into our homes and personal spaces, a reflection of how much we need to maintain the deep connection we feel to the natural world.

Environmental Integration

One of the great benefits of exercising outside is the experience of connecting to the natural world around you. This process of connecting mentally and physically to nature is what I call environmental integration. Awareness of your environment keeps you safe on the trail; it also promotes a feeling of "oneness" with the natural world around you. Nature becomes both a guide and a companion.

In Outdoor Fitness, you learn to adapt the laws of nature to your workout and your mindset. You learn to "go with the flow." You don't conquer a mountain, battle a tricky path, or fight your way through tall grass. This approach puts you at odds with your environment and leads to rigidity, tension, and stress. Instead, you let go and relax. Like a bird in the wind or a fish in a stream, your body and mind flow freely with the forces of nature, the elements and terrain you encounter, gravity itself.

The key to environmental integration is right in front of your nose. Actually, it *is* your nose, as well as your eyes and ears, your hands and feet, and even your inner "gut," or instinct. When you're exercising outdoors, you'll have the chance to be in constant sensory contact with nature. There's so much to absorb:

- **Visual:** Lightness, darkness, textures, colors, movement, scenery, sky, objects
- **Auditory:** Chirping birds, water flowing, lapping waves, cracking twigs, rustling leaves, the sound of your own breathing
- **Olfactory:** Scent of trees, flowers, rain, the sea, dirt, animals
- **Intuitive:** Following a hunch, having a deep feeling about something, relying on your inner resources

Tuning in to your senses—including your powerful intuition—will deepen and expand your experience of working out. You'll feel confident, connected, and part of a much bigger world—the natural world.

Reading the Terrain

One of the most practical ways you'll use environmental integration is by learning to "read" your environment. No more jogging with your head down! Exercising in the outdoors means you need to be constantly observing your surroundings: looking ahead, noting twists and turns in the trail or angles of slope in the road. Watching out for obstacles and changes to the terrain itself, from gravel to pavement to dirt; wet spots on the sidewalk; roots, rocks, and sticks on the ground. By reading your environment, you give mind and body time to anticipate and adapt to what's coming, so you're prepared to move over terrain safely and without wasting effort. Reading your environment also keeps you connected to what's around you. When you're scanning ahead for changes in terrain, you're also experiencing sights, scents, and sounds that stimulate and inspire you.

Keys to Integrating with Your Environment

- Tune in to your surroundings.
- Feel the terrain underfoot.
- Relax and feel the pull of gravity.
- Notice the colors and textures.
- Take in the sounds around you.
- Feel the breeze brush your skin.
- Smell the aroma in the air.
- Trust and listen to your internal voice.
- Close your eyes occasionally during an exercise. This helps enhance your other senses.

Physical Strength and Skill

Physical conditioning is the basis of what brings everyone to Outdoor Fitness, and it is the core of the program itself. To grow stronger and more agile. To run farther and faster. To trim and slim and tone our shapes. The physical components of Outdoor Fitness are muscular strength and endurance, cardiovascular conditioning, and flexibility and balance. Two other important aspects of the program are kinesthetic awareness and proprioceptive awareness, skills that bridge physical and mental spheres and allow the whole body to function more confidently and efficiently in its environment.

Muscular Strength and Endurance

In Outdoor Fitness, you'll gain muscular strength and endurance in every workout by using my original Base Moves and Signature Moves. The health benefits of resistance training are clear: Building muscular strength and endurance can prevent and reverse the effects of aging in both men and women. These two types of muscular training are both critical to your well-rounded workout and your overall health. Muscular strength is the ability of a muscle to lift a heavy object or exert maximum force over a short amount of time. Muscular strength training involves high resistance and low repetitions. One to two sets of 8 to 12 repetitions per set will increase strength and definition. Muscular endurance is the ability to exert force over and over again for an extended period of time. Muscular endurance training uses low to medium resistance and high repetitions. One or two sets for an extended period of time, such as a full minute, will increase endurance and tone.

Cardiovascular Conditioning

Improving cardiovascular fitness is another central objective of Outdoor Fitness. You'll keep busy with everything from fast-paced walks in the park to loops along a rural path, from hill sprints to drills on an athletic field. Progress in cardiovascular conditioning is easy to spot. Maybe you're starting out the program as a walker—in a few weeks, you'll need to jog to break a sweat. Maybe you're already a runner—get ready for your pace to increase and your body to feel like it was born to run! Whatever your starting fitness level, cardiovascular fitness will be one of the key

Concentric and Eccentric

The contraction phase of an exercise is also called the concentric phase, while the relaxation phase is the eccentric phase. In a pull-up, the lifting phase is concentric and the lowering phase is eccentric. In a squat, the lowering phase is eccentric and the return phase is concentric. Why does this matter? Coordinating your breath with your exercise protects your body. You should exhale during the tough part, the contraction, or concentric, phase, and inhale during the easier, or eccentric, phase. Regulating breath and movement this way alleviates stress on the heart and keeps blood pressure from increasing.

There are plenty of options for props to assist you in muscular strength and endurance training. The best tool when working in the outdoors is your own body! This program's outdoor workouts rely on your body's own weight and gravity for building muscular strength and endurance.

measurements of your progress.

Rate of Perceived Exertion, or RPE, is the most important measuring tool you'll use day to day in your outdoor workouts. This is a subjective, self-determined measurement of your muscular, cardiovascular, and psychological fatigue. RPE measures your heart rate—and your exertion level—by asking you to assess your own fatigue in the moment. Monitoring and controlling your RPE helps you make the most of your workout time: By managing your exertion, you burn fat and calories and build muscle more efficiently. Many times throughout your workouts, you'll be prompted to gauge your RPE. There is no wrong answer—whatever you feel in that moment is the right response. Using the RPE Level of Exertion Scale, check in with yourself during a workout. If you can carry on a conversation with ease, then you're probably not working hard enough. If you can carry on a conversation but find yourself not really wanting to, then you are beginning to maximize your workout.

Tips for Exercising Using Body Weight

- Do each exercise in a slow and controlled manner; don't let momentum do the work for you.
- Use the core of your body for added strength and support.
- Pay equal attention to both eccentric and concentric phases of the movement.
- Always use proper breathing. Exhale during the exertion phase of the exercise.
- Connect internally—mentally, visually, and kinesthetically—with the muscle groups you're working.
- Use gravity to your advantage.

RPE Level of Exertion Scale

1. Very weak
2. Weak
3. Somewhat moderate
4. Moderate
5. Somewhat strong (can still easily carry on a conversation)
6. Strong
7. Very strong (aerobic zone; can talk but don't feel like it)
8. Even stronger
9. Very, very strong (anaerobic zone; can't talk at all)
10. Maximum (anaerobic zone)

There are two cardio training zones you'll need to know about to manage your workouts for maximum benefit.

Aerobic conditioning takes place when your body is working with oxygen. This type of training makes up the bulk of your cardiovascular work. The American College of Sports Medicine recommends 30 minutes of aerobic conditioning on most days, meaning five or more days per week. Aerobic conditioning improves your body's ability to transport oxygen and to clear carbon dioxide, and it improves endurance.

Anaerobic conditioning takes place when your body is working without oxygen because of the intensity of your exertion. Anaerobic conditioning builds muscular power, strength, and speed, and it is an important part of your routine. You might include anaerobic conditioning in your workouts one to two times per week for general conditioning, and up to two to three times per week for high-performance athletes.

Flexibility and Balance

In each workout, you'll spend time working on both flexibility and balance. Your warm-up and cooldown are prime times to concentrate on flexibility. You will also find flexibility exercises and stretches in chapter 4. Becoming more flexible aids performance, prevents injury, increases circulation, lengthens tight muscles, and removes waste from your system. It's important to warm up before you stretch so that you slowly raise your heart rate, which will increase circulation and oxygenation of muscles, speed up nerve impulses, and warm and lubricate muscles, ligaments, and joints. Warming up before stretching not only makes your muscles more pliable, it protects your joints by lubricating them with your body's own synovial fluid, which nourishes cartilage and keeps joints stable.

Balance is an aspect of fitness that is so often overlooked. As we age, we are all at risk of falling and breaking bones—and poor fitness and balance skills make us more vulnerable. Many of my exercises include elements that challenge your balance skills. Balance requires strength, body awareness, and focus. Working on balance brings together the mental and the physical, connecting mind and muscle in a single task.

Kinesthetic Awareness

Kinesthetic awareness is your body's comprehension of its place in its environment, and its ability to move through that environment fluidly—with control, ease, and grace. To understand kinesthetic awareness, think about the way a cat moves through its environment.

Balanced, agile, and surefooted, a cat moves gracefully and purposefully over all types of terrain. From the way it knows just how much energy it needs to leap to the top of a wall to the way it manages to land on its four feet when it falls to the ground, a cat always has its bearings. This is kinesthetic awareness in action.

Human beings have this ability, too. It's something we're born with, but unfortunately it's something that often goes dormant within us as we age and our lives become sedentary. The good news is that your kinesthetic awareness is just sitting inside you, waiting to be cultivated!

Developing kinesthetic awareness is one of the most important goals of Outdoor Fitness, one that brings the body, the mind, and the emotions into play, asking them to work in harmony. Your brain and your body must work together to adjust quickly to the unpredictable and ever-changing conditions and terrain. Outdoor Fitness training demands that you use your kinesthetic power and rewards you by developing this power quickly and to a degree that you may otherwise not have experienced.

You'll find that this is a skill that affects the movements you do in all parts of your life, from getting into and out of your car and playing with your kids to playing a game of pickup basketball and competing in your local 10K race.

Proprioceptive Awareness

Now think about your hands. They're remarkable, aren't they? Think about all that you do with your hands in a single hour of a single day. Your hands react instinctively, with great precision, to hundreds of tasks and actions in the span of a single hour. Your proprioceptive awareness is best demonstrated in your hands.

Proprioceptive awareness is a close cousin to kinesthetic awareness. Here's how they are related: Proprioceptors are nerve endings located in the muscles and their tendons. These nerve endings respond to tension, providing all the sensory information your brain and body need to be aware of itself in its environment—that is, to be kinesthetically aware. Proprioceptors are the neurological messengers that enable kinesthetic awareness. Proprioceptive awareness itself is a fine-tuned spatial sensitivity. It enables you to manage uneven terrain and keep from turning an ankle.

Proprioception Exercise

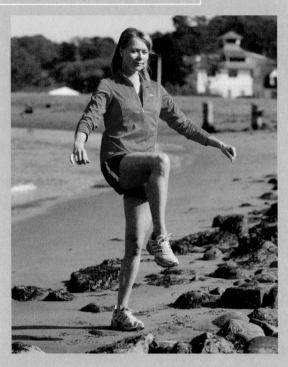 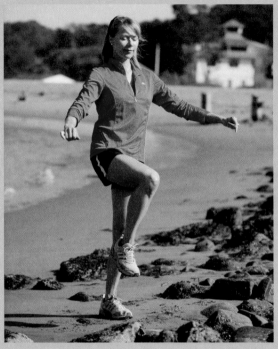

Stand on flat ground, extending your arms comfortably for balance and your hands within your peripheral vision.

Lift your right knee up and hold for 5 to 30 seconds. Don't worry if you are wobbly; just relax and connect with your center of mass, right below your navel. Repeat with the other leg.

At some point, if the exercise becomes too easy, you can try it with your eyes closed.

Work on increasing your time.

Feel through Your Feet

Foot sensitivity is a key to developing both kinesthetic and proprioceptive awareness. In the outdoors, the terrain and ground texture are constantly changing. One of your goals in Outdoor Fitness is to develop your foot sensitivity so that it is on par with the sensitivity in your hands. This may sound impossible, but it's not! Your feet are the first, and most important, contact you make with the earth. Like your hands, you have more than 7,000 nerve endings in each foot. Your feet are capable of receiving a remarkable amount of sensory information, enabling your whole body and mind to react to changing environmental conditions. Prepare to become sure-footed like you've never imagined you could be—especially on uneven and ever-changing terrain! Interestingly enough, a study conducted by researchers from the Oregon Research Institute investigated the health effects of walking on cobblestone-like surfaces. They discovered that walking on such uneven surfaces significantly lowered blood pressure and improved balance. Reflexologists believe that uneven terrain can stimulate acupressure points in the soles of the feet to relieve pain, improve sleep patterns, and enhance overall well-being.

Mental and Emotional Power

You'll hear me remind you many times throughout your workouts: Thoughts are things. The impact of our mental and emotional selves on our physical selves cannot be overestimated. Thoughts and feelings have a direct physiological impact on our bodies. Here's a quick example: Think about an ice-cold, tart cherry. See it in your mind's eye, and imagine the chill in your fingertips from grasping it. Now imagine popping it in your mouth and rolling it around on your

tongue. Cold and smooth. Now imagine biting into it. Did your mouth begin to water? If a simple thought can do that to your tongue, imagine what negative, anxiety-producing thoughts can do to your body!

There is great power in this relationship between mind, emotions, and body. Elite athletes know that mental attitude accounts for 80 percent or more of performance. Visualizing a goal, and using positive self-talk to reinforce your abilities, can get you where you want to go—top of the hill, last set of squats, one last push-up. So, too, negative thoughts and anxious feelings can sabotage all your efforts. Harnessing the power of your mind and your emotions can transform your workouts, and your life, too.

The Five Beat Rule

Negative thoughts put direct stress on the body, particularly the central nervous system. Your mind races, adrenalin flows through the bloodstream, and your heart rate can increase up to five beats per minute. Conversely, soothing, calming thoughts can lower your heart rate by five beats. It all comes down to a choice—what do you *choose* to focus on?

Marissa, Age 26

Rather than being full of motivation, I was full of excuses. I was frustrated because the gym I'd belonged to for the past three years was just another bill that needed to be paid. I was overweight, undermotivated (often sleeping until noon), and incredibly scattered—physically, mentally, and emotionally. Even my driving was unfit! Little did I know that a phone call to Tina Vindum's Outdoor Fitness would literally change my life, create a new me, and be tantamount in fulfilling my dreams of becoming an actress.

It was through Outdoor Fitness that I learned to take responsibility for my health, fitness, and well-being. It's been three months since I started the program, and I've made a complete transformation physically, personally, and in my daily habits. I now look forward to rising early and getting positively charged through trees, water, sun, rain—real life that fuels my life!

The demands of Outdoor Fitness require mental focus and emotional control. You are rewarded with increased mental acuity, concentration, and self-awareness. Self-reflection and even self-discovery are benefits of Outdoor Fitness that often surprise people: So many of my clients start this program seeking the physical results but find the mental and emotional results to be the most profound and exciting changes in their lives.

As your mental focus builds, you will find greater power to influence and improve performance by controlling and directing your thoughts and emotions.

Becoming emotionally fit can be as liberating and health promoting as physical fitness. You'll discover new avenues for personal growth, make positive changes to your life, increase your ability to trust, and find a deep sense of gratitude within yourself for many things in your life, including the ability to be healthy. You'll begin to discover your mental and emotional power out on the trail. What you'll soon learn is that you can take this power off the trail and into your life, helping you to navigate the bumps and twists that life brings with grace and inner calm.

CHAPTER 2

Mental Fitness and the BodyMind Connection: Reaching Your Mental and Emotional Peak

Athletes know that mental focus is as much a part of training and skill as physical prowess. Working out in the outdoors requires that you concentrate and adapt as you adjust to new conditions and changing terrain. Outdoor Fitness makes mental focus and acuity training a cornerstone of its program. Within the BodyMind connection, mindfulness, concentration, and emotional power techniques are integrated with the physical elements of the workouts to create a true whole health and fitness program.

Just like our bodies get in a rut from inactivity or the same old gym routine, our minds also fall into unhealthful, limiting habits. We fall prey to the same emotional triggers, the same negative self-talk, the same distractions, day after day. Outdoor Fitness gives you a chance to transform your emotional landscape

and literally rewire your brain. Deepening mental focus brings with it tremendous freedom. The vast power of the mind can shape our lives, enhance our health and well-being, and create success and achievement. Developing your mental focus and emotional control will bring your workout and sports performance to new levels. It also has the power to transform your life beyond the trail.

What Is BodyMind?

Here's some news that might surprise you: The BodyMind connection is not a mystical, otherworldly, nebulous thing. It really exists—and you don't need to be a yogi to access it! There is now scientific evidence to support a centuries-old philosophy: The body and the mind are not two separate spheres, but they are

Allison, Age 35

Allison was training for the trip of a lifetime, an expedition to climb the highest peak in North America: Mount McKinley, at 20,320 feet, in Alaska's Denali National Park. The expedition would take anywhere from 17 to 30 days, and she would be the lone female on the team. She approached me with her goal, and I was excited at the chance to train her.

We spent a lot of time working on her strength and endurance, but the combination of fierce weather, high altitude, and the 60-pound pack she would be required to haul meant Allison would not only need to be in the best physical shape of her life, she'd also need to be in top mental shape.

Concentration skills were essential for her, especially during those clutch moments when she needed to perform on the spot. Mental focus creates the ability to consistently perform well under pressure.

Upon returning from her successful climb, Allison was elated. "Even when I knew I had to perform or the whole expedition was in danger, my training helped me directly concentrate on the task at hand," she said. "I was completely committed to the climb at all times. Mental focus training made all the difference!"

in fact deeply entwined. In the 1970s, American scientist Candace Pert made a historic discovery that would have a profound impact on our understanding of both mind and body. She identified molecules whose purpose was to unlock brain cells and allow morphine and other opiates to enter the cells. Uncovering the nexus where mind, matter, and emotions collide, Pert had quite literally found the key to a tangible link between the body and the mind.

Since then, scientists have discovered these "unlocking" molecules, called neuropeptide receptors, throughout the body. The result of these discoveries has been the identification of a network that links the brain, the endocrine system, the immune system, and the nervous system in a relationship where each communicates with the other. Gone is the old notion that the brain "controls" the body. Through Dr. Pert's research, we now know that both our mental and physical selves—our minds and our matter—cooperate in making our bodies work. We also know that our emotions, as Dr. Pert explains, are a kind of "nexus between our mind and our matter, carrying messages back and forth and influencing both." Essentially this means that when we think negative thoughts, we release certain chemicals that weaken both our physical health and psychological well-being; when we consciously create positive thoughts, we can literally boost our health—in both our minds and our bodies. This is what I mean when I say you can rewire your brain through exercise. The exercise makes you feel good, which in turn creates more positive thoughts.

So what does the BodyMind connection mean for you and your health and fitness? As your Outdoor Fitness coach, I care about your whole body and your total health. I don't just care about getting your body into shape—I care about helping you shape up your BodyMind. Mental, emotional, and physical wellness are equal partners in Outdoor Fitness, just as they are in your BodyMind. Remember, more often than not, we humans aren't motivated by rational thought but by our emotions.

Rather than taking on a boot camp mentality of discipline and butt kicking, I'd like you to find flow and ease, where exercise comes naturally and without effort so you are drawn to feeling good—physically, mentally, and emotionally.

Tears on the Trail

Emotional experiences and life events are stored physiologically in your body. When you work deep in your body to

Mood and Posture

The relationship between mood and posture provides an illuminating glimpse into the connection between body and mind. Body positioning can instantly affect our emotions and our mood. When we are depressed or sad, we instinctively look down at the ground. When we try to hold back tears, we automatically turn our faces upward, as if to keep the tears from falling.

Here's a quick exercise that illustrates the power of this connection:

- Stand in an idle position, with your shoulders slouched and your eyes focused down toward the ground. Take shallow breaths. How do you feel?
- Now stand in a position of strength and positive emotion. Lift your chin up. Turn your eyes toward the sky. Smile. Breathe deeply. How do you feel now?

release tensions and challenge your body to new physical heights, this can often bring about emotions. This is normal—in fact, it's a good, healthy thing. I think of it as a side benefit of your Outdoor Fitness training. You're going to learn a great deal about controlling and clearing your emotions, channeling your thoughts and feelings. Many people experience intense feelings and even cry—I call this "tears on the trail" because it's so common! Remember that emotions are natural, embrace your feelings in the moment, and take time later on to reflect on what you discovered in your workout. The key is to eliminate those emotions that no longer serve you and replace them with emotions that do.

Mental Focus Is the Key to BodyMind Health

In Outdoor Fitness, you cultivate mental focus just as you develop physical strength and endurance. It's a component to all the workouts, a skill to develop and hone, a tool to spur you to greater achievements and better health for your BodyMind. What is mental focus? Simply, it's the ability to concentrate on the task at hand, to put your attention on the present moment without interruption from internal chatter or external distractions.

Another way to express this is in terms of mindfulness. When you are mindful, your mind is full of *this moment*. You're not planning your next workout or replaying a conversation from earlier in the day. You're not worrying about what your boss will think of your latest brief or beating yourself up for not running an eight-minute mile. You are immersed, simply and completely, in *now*. In a very real sense, mindfulness is the mental equivalent of kinesthetic awareness. Just as your body is attuned to its moment-to-moment environment, your mind is aware of and occupied in a moment-to-moment consciousness.

The benefits of mindfulness, and of mental focus training, go way beyond a more peaceful and effective workout. The positive effects of mindfulness impact all aspects of your life. You experience:

• decrease in stress
• increase in your sense of well-being
• feeling more engaged at work and in relationships
• better social interaction
• more energy
• less anxiety
• greater emotional control
• better mood
• greater ability to concentrate
• greater productivity

Mental Imagery: Visualize Your Best Self

One of the best ways to prepare for a challenging workout is to fill your mind with uplifting, positive images. This is a great exercise to do during your warm-up. You can also use imagery exercises during a specific exercise or during a cardio session.

Close your eyes. Imagine yourself performing well during your workout. Feel your lungs filling with air, your breath originating with the deep exhale of the diaphragm. Feel your head held upright, your eyes forward, taking in the path ahead and the beauty of the scenery. See yourself moving confidently over the terrain. Imagine yourself feeling energized, confident, and powerful. See yourself gliding over the trail. Do you feel your muscles begin to twitch? Good. Now put one foot in front of the other and repeat. Literally step into the picture and feel how easily your body and mind begin to flow as you move into your workout.

Challenges to Mindfulness

Just as flexibility and strength are acquired skills, so too is mental focus. It's not always easy to be mindful in our world. Distractions that take you out of the moment lurk everywhere. In a workout, just as in our lives, distractions can be both internal and external. External distractions during a workout are legion and varied: other people talking, traffic, animals, activity on the street, or scenery on the trail. Internal distractions are sometimes less obvious but are no less potent challenges to mental focus. Our self-talk—the running commentary that we all carry in our minds—is a constant challenge to mindfulness. Self-talk often becomes habitual and rote. We think the same negative thoughts over and over again, sabotaging our mood and performance. So many of our negative thoughts have been with us for years, chipping away at our self-esteem and our belief in our abilities. With mindfulness training, you can replace these negative thoughts with a new, positive set of thoughts and beliefs about yourself. You get to create a new, fresh set of thoughts, images, and beliefs about who you are and what you're capable of.

Learning to be mindful begins with understanding the ways our brains are *not* in the moment. The simple PMJ exercise that follows is one you'll return to again and again in your workouts, and it can help erase distractions by identifying thoughts that pass through your brain, then releasing them. You can use this exercise during a workout or in a meditation session.

PMJ Exercise: Plans, Memories, Judgments

All your thoughts can be broken down into three basic types:

Plans: Goals, lists, plans for the future ("What's for dinner?" "What do I really want to do with my career?" "I need to get my car inspected.")

Memories: Thoughts from or about the past (yesterday's tense conversation with your boyfriend, last year's raucous holiday party, the fight you had with your mom before leaving for college).

Judgments: Thoughts, feelings, and opinions ("My butt is saggy." "I hated that movie last night." "My boss is a terror.")

This exercise is simple and so effective at dismissing all these distractions to mindfulness. To begin, let your mind go to whatever thoughts it wants. When a thought arises, identify it for yourself as a plan, a memory, or a judgment. Once you've identified the thought, release it. Poof! Just like that, it's gone. When you find yourself having difficulty clearing your mind, ask yourself: "What is my next thought?" Notice what happens? Poof! Just like that your mental screen is clear. Asking this question brings you right back to the present.

Thoughts Are Things

Human beings are incredible—and unique—in the power that our thoughts have to shape who we are. We have the ability to become who we *think* we are and to do what we *think* we can do. Our thoughts are incredibly powerful. If, while trekking up a steep hill, you think, "This is way too hard for me; I'm not

Meditation Can Make You Happier and Healthier

In a remarkable collaborative study between the Dalai Lama and some of the country's finest neuroscientists, researchers found that meditation and mindfulness training enhance the brain's ability to eliminate distressing feelings in favor of optimistic, upbeat feelings and thoughts. In their article in the peer-reviewed journal *Psychosomatic Medicine*, Dr. Richard Davidson and Dr. Jon Kabat-Zinn also reported that training in mindfulness meditation also supports and strengthens the immune system.

Tina's Story: Rabbit Trails

I first learned about the power of my thoughts while jogging on my favorite wooded trail in Mill Valley. One moment, I'd be moving along at a steady clip, running smoothly and getting the job done. Then, the next moment, I found myself moving at a snail's pace, unsteady, head down and in deep thought. Sometimes my thoughts were about the past and some painful mishap. I'd find myself replaying the tape of this past event, as if I could somehow change the plot. Most often, though, the thoughts were about the future, and "what if" questions about things that will never happen. I call these fear-based, emotionally charged, anxiety-producing thoughts "rabbit trails."

I became frustrated with the unevenness of my workout and the way that my habitual thoughts affected how I felt and performed. In looking for a way to get beyond this roadblock, I started to backtrack. When I found myself way down the path of a rabbit trail, I would follow that trail right back to the initial thought that started the whole sequence. Wow! It was an enormous eye-opener for me. I soon realized I'd start on one thought, like an ex-boyfriend, and I'd travel from thought to thought, scene to scene, like a rabbit hopping from point to point in a zigzag. I was able to mentally peg the precise moment and section of the actual trail where the first thought had arisen—and I saw how these thoughts changed my performance. Wearing a heart rate monitor, I also noticed that my heart rate would rise an average of five beats per minute. To top it off, I'd create a downer mood for myself that could last for hours.

I learned to track my thoughts back to what I call "trigger thoughts." These are thoughts that do not serve me or my well-being. Over time, I learned to keep my thoughts clean, clear, and focused on the task at hand. I'd remind myself, "This is not the time, and if I need to think about that, it'll be there waiting for me when I get back." Instead, I learned to fully integrate with the terrain and the environment around me, feeling happy, powerful, and fully focused on the present moment.

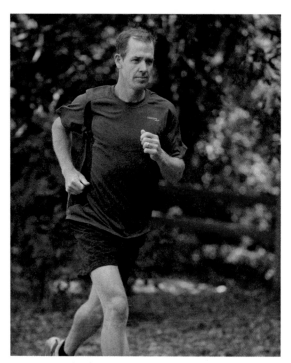

Run strong, yet relaxed

Intensity, Concentration, and Relaxation: 3 Ways to Focus

Great athletes know the power of the mind to influence performance. They know the hallmarks of success aren't just brawn or speed, but inevitably are concentration, intensity, and relaxation— each of which requires mental focus to achieve. When you're working out, especially when you're exercising outdoors, you need to be able to draw on all three types of mental focus skills. You practice concentration in your moment-to-moment focus on the task at hand, blocking out distractions. You practice intensity by your mental commitment to the exercise you're involved in, and by giving yourself the mental stimulation you need to complete your task. You practice relaxation by performing your workouts without tension and anxiety. Intensity, concentration, and relaxation are learned skills. You train for these skills just as you train for strength and speed.

There are several simple techniques that you can rely on during a workout to help find your mental focus and that combination of intensity, concentration, and relaxation:

strong enough for this. I'll never make it to the top," you will prove yourself right. If, on the other hand, you think, "This is a tough one. I'm going to give this my best shot, dig in, and make it to the top," you will also prove yourself right. That's how quickly and easily our thoughts have the power to influence reality, to become things. In that moment, you choose the outcome by choosing your thoughts. This is why positive self-talk is such an important skill, in your workouts and in your life off the trail.

- **Give your mind a warm-up.** Familiarize yourself with the components of your workout and its purpose. Just as your body needs time to prepare for the physical task ahead, your mind needs warm-up time to acclimate to what is to come.

- **Pay attention to your inner voice.** You know how common negative self-talk is and how damaging it can be. Gently acknowledge any negative judgment as it arises and replace it with a positive affirmation. As you breathe, think: "Positive in, negative out."

- **Use your environment to relax.** Open yourself up to your surroundings. Nature is a powerful relaxation tool. Feel through your feet. Listen to the sound of leaves rustling. Smell, taste, and feel the crashing of the sea nearby.

- **Remind yourself of mindfulness!** Remember the simple truth of mindfulness. Allow your mind to be full of the moment. Practice a quick PMJ exercise to rid yourself of distracting thoughts. Use a positive moving mantra—*I am strong! I feel alive!*—to keep yourself in the present.

- **Smile.** Definitely the simplest technique, and maybe the most potent, the physical act of smiling has an immediate and positive effect on your body and your mind. You can't help but feel better when you smile. (Try it now.) Use this when you feel you need a boost.

- **Use power words.** Finding a few meaningful and inspiring words to use during clutch moments of your workout can help you ramp up your intensity, focus your concentration, or relax your body. "Dig deep!" "Low and slow." Create your own power words to help trigger your mental focus.

Flashlight Technique

Jim Taylor, a San Francisco–based sports psychologist who has worked with world-class and professional athletes, uses this technique with his clients. This mental focus technique alternates between peripheral vision and pinpoint visual focus, much like the broad and narrow beams of a good flashlight. It's ideal for cardio and trail work. As you're walking or running, continuously switch between your peripheral vision, or "broad focus," to "take in the whole picture" and your pinpoint, or "narrow focus," to zero in on the center of your immediate view. Peripheral vision allows your mind to read the broad picture, and narrow focus allows you to hone in on your target area for accuracy. This practice keeps your mind engaged constantly with its moment-to-moment surroundings, broad and narrow. It also challenges your mental flexibility and concentration as you continually reset your attention.

HeartBrain Technique

Did you know that you can actually think with your heart? It's true! Neurocardiologists in the mid-1990s made a startling discovery: There is actually a "brain" inside the heart. The so-called HeartBrain refers to a set of nerve cells, neurotransmitters, and support cells that together have highly computational abilities. The HeartBrain can learn, remember, and form responses, and it does so independently of the brain in your head. This may sound like science fiction, but think for a moment about how we identify with our hearts versus our heads.

Let's start with language. Think about the way we talk about ourselves and others. When someone displays bravery, is determined and resilient, we say: "He's got heart." When we're doing well in a sport or activity, we say: "I was playing out of my head."

Now try this simple exercise. Point to yourself.

Did you point to your head? I bet not. I'm guessing you pointed to your chest.

See the pattern emerging? When we think of ourselves, we think through our hearts. Getting "out of our heads" is synonymous with success, flow, and working smoothly and successfully at the task at hand. Getting out of our heads also means getting into someplace else—our hearts, our core being. Now that you know your heart has the power to lead you, you can let your mind take a backseat now and then. Remind yourself to literally "lead with your heart" when you're on the trail.

Slashing Your Stress Level in the Great Outdoors

As a culture, we are used to accepting stress as part of life. What we don't often recognize are the physical effects of allowing stress to accompany us throughout our days. Your entire (BodyMind) system is directly affected by the physical, mental, and emotional stresses of your daily life. Spending time outside enjoying nature is one of the most basic ways to help reduce your stress level and boost your immune system, a critical aspect to overall health and well-being. Studies show that our environment contributes up to 70 percent of our stress. Unfortunately, most people spend over 90 percent of their waking hours indoors. In today's automated world of technology and urban living, our bonds with nature have been fractured, and people are more rushed, stressed, overweight, and depressed then ever before. Seldom do people find themselves enjoying the outdoors and reaping the health benefits of serenity and calm that nature has to offer.

Take a moment to think about peace and tranquility. Really sit back and allow yourself to meditate on what serenity looks and feels like to you. What kinds of images came to your mind? Did you think about watching television, or shopping, or traffic? Highly unlikely! For most people, thinking about tranquility and peace brings forth images of nature. Maybe you imagined yourself in a mountain meadow, or alongside the crashing surf. Nature soothes our mind and calms our senses. This is a deeply rooted comfort. For as long as we have been evolving as a species, Mother Nature has been nurturing us by helping us to maintain our psychological, physical, and emotional health.

Simply put, real relaxation isn't found on the couch. Some people think relaxation and stress reduction consist of lying back in an easy chair and watching TV, or having a cocktail with friends, or perhaps taking in a movie. All this may seem and even feel relaxing—but there is a big difference between this kind of relaxation and the ability to reach a much deeper and revitalizing state of relaxation. Regular exercise, with attention to your mental and physical fitness—especially in the outdoors, surrounded by nature's calming effects—can bring you deep, restorative relaxation. This restorative relaxation is the immune-system-boosting, stress-reducing kind—the kind you'll never get on the couch, or even at the gym.

Use the following exercises when you find yourself feeling tense, anxious, and stressed. These exercises can be especially useful at the outset of a workout, when you're trying to shake off the effects of your busy day.

Body Clench

- Clench your fists, arms, chest, abs, glutes, and legs.
- Hold for a count of 10.
- Slowly release, and let your whole body go completely limp. Repeat 3 or more times.

Fist Clench with Diaphragmatic Breath

- Clench your fists tightly as you take a deep diaphragmatic breath, and hold it for a count of 10.
- Exhale thoroughly and completely, as you let your body go limp.

A Checklist for the 10 Aspects of Mental Fitness

As you think about all of what goes into rewiring your brain for exercise, achieving BodyMind balance and health, use this checklist as a way to make sure you are tapping into all the ways to stay connected and boost your positive thoughts and emotions. If you're hitting all the points, you're hitting a perfect score.

- ☐ **Mindfulness.** Stay in the moment.
- ☐ **Self-talk.** Keep self-talk positive. Let go of negative thoughts.
- ☐ **Concentration.** Keep your attention on your exercise/task for the duration.
- ☐ **Intensity.** Perform at the level you need to so that you can gain the rewards you're seeking.
- ☐ **Relaxation.** Exercise without tension or anxiety.
- ☐ **Stress relief.** Exercise to eliminate stress, finding peace and tranquility.
- ☐ **Emotional balance.** Observe and respect your emotions as they arise. Let them go so that you are not being controlled by them.
- ☐ **"Rabbit trails."** Avoid negative thought patterns and identify your "trigger thoughts" and emotions.
- ☐ **Visualization.** Imagine your best self.
- ☐ **Reflection.** Take time to think about what you're learning. I always say self-reflection is synonymous with personal growth.

TIP: To help find a rhythm of deep breathing and positive emotion, try using this mantra as you inhale and exhale: "Positive in, negative out."

CHAPTER 3

Getting Ready

This chapter is all about getting you outfitted—body and mind—to begin your Outdoor Fitness program. For a happier, healthier, well-balanced life, it's important to think about what your goals really are. My questions will help you zero in on your health, fitness, and social and emotional goals. You'll also take a look at your schedule to examine how you spend your time and energy and figure out a way to fit in fitness. With a schedule in place, your goals become achievable, manageable milestones to work toward every day.

Next you'll learn all about selecting locations and ways to stay safe while exploring and enjoying nature. The outdoors is full of possibilities for fun, excitement, and exertion like you've never experienced in a workout program. The natural world is also full of challenges and potential hazards you must understand in order to stay safe and make the best use of your remarkable environment. From weather and climate conditions to pesky flora and fauna, you'll get the rundown on how to dress for the weather, how to navigate your environment, how to train safely to avoid injury, and what to do in the unlikely event that an injury does happen.

Setting Goals

People come to Outdoor Fitness with a wide range of goals. Part of being a total health program means Outdoor Fitness can accommodate many types of goals—physical, mental, and social; competitive; illness-related; restorative; and more. Maybe you have a weight-loss target you'd like to achieve at the end of 12 weeks. Maybe there is a 10K road race you'd like to run. Maybe you're working to avoid or eliminate a diagnosis of type 2 diabetes or high blood pressure. Maybe you have a special event coming up—a wedding or a class reunion—and you want to walk in feeling trim and fit and looking great. Goal setting is a very personal, individual process—and your goals are your own. What's important is that you set them, monitor them, and praise yourself when you accomplish them.

The Power of 3

3 seconds: The time it takes to make a decision. Making a clear decision about what you'd like to achieve is the most powerful step you can take in realizing your goals.

3 days: The time it takes to get "on the rails"—and ride the track in the direction you'd like to go.

3 weeks: The time it takes to create a routine. Now you are clearly living and feeling the Outdoor Fitness lifestyle.

3 months: The time it takes to *own* that new routine. There are numerous studies that show in order to completely change a behavior and set a new one requires 90 days. Just think—only 12 weeks to own your new life with style!

Strategies for Goal Setting

Outdoor Fitness is not just about a firmer butt and better biceps; it's about health, fitness, and well-being, and creating a better lifestyle—a life with *style!* However, it takes more than just fat loss and firm muscles. For a happier, healthier, well-balanced life, it's important to create goals in all areas of our lives. So let's take a moment to explore what your goals in life *really* are, then *decide* to follow through.

One of the challenges of goal setting is keeping your aspirations specific, reasonable, and attainable. You set yourself up for frustration if you decide you must lose 20 pounds in a month or run 5 miles after a couple of weeks. A strategy that can help is to divide your goals into short-term and long-term goals. Short-term goals are things like increasing cardiovascular fitness, losing body fat, reducing stress, and improving flexibility. Long-term goals are things like running a marathon, losing 30 pounds, and reducing the risk of heart disease.

Another strategy is to think beyond the obvious. Okay, so you know you want to lose some weight and trim your waist. What are the social or emotional goals that accompany your physical ones? What are your whole health aspirations?

Use the following questionnaire to help you determine your goals.

Goal-Setting Questionnaire and Commitment Contract

Find a quiet place, free from distractions. Unplug the phone, close the e-mail screen, and focus . . . on you!

1. To begin the process of setting goals, take a moment to jot down what you are currently *dissatisfied* with in your life. For example: "I am tired of passing on social events because I don't have the energy to go." Or, "I have had it with carrying around this extra 20 pounds!"

_____

_____

2. *Specifically,* what are your:

Health goals? Example: "I would like to reduce my cholesterol by 20 percent."

_____

Fitness goals? Example: "I will exercise for at least 40 minutes every morning."

_____

Psychological goals? Example: "I will reduce my stress levels and increase my mental focus abilities." _____

Social (family/friends) goals? Example: "I will spend at least two afternoons a week hiking with a friend."_____

_____

3. *Why* are these goals important to you? How will you feel when you accomplish them?

Health: _____

_____

Fitness:_____

_____

Psychological:_____

_____

Social: _____

_____

4. Have you set these goals for yourself in the past? Did you follow through? Yes ___ No ___ If you answered "yes," explain how you were able to accomplish them._____

_____

_____

_____

If you answered "no," explain what got in the way of accomplishing your goals. Be honest with yourself! _____

_____

_____

_____

5. In order to reach your goals, what is required of you? _____

_____

_____

_____

6. Using a scale from one (low) to 5 (high), how would you rate your current physical, mental, and emotional condition?:

Cardiovascular	**1 2 3 4 5**
Muscle strength and endurance	**1 2 3 4 5**
Flexibility	**1 2 3 4 5**
Balance and coordination	**1 2 3 4 5**
Mental focus	**1 2 3 4 5**
Emotional well-being	**1 2 3 4 5**
Social interaction	**1 2 3 4 5**

7. What areas require more attention from you?_____

_____

_____

_____

8. Are you committed to eating healthfully? _____ If so, how could you improve your diet?

_____

_____

9. How much time are you willing to devote to your lifestyle program?_____

_____

_____

10. Would a new lifestyle program improve your relationships? _____How?_____

_____

_____

_____

How about your work? _____

_____

_____

_____

11. Looking again at your health, fitness, and wellness goals in number 2 above:
Why are these goals important for you to achieve? _____

_____

_____

_____

How would you *feel* if you accomplished these goals? _____

_____

_____

_____

How would you *feel* if you did not reach these goals? _____

_____

_____

_____

12. Take a moment to create your exercise schedule:

Day	Time Start/Time Finish
Sunday	_____
Monday	_____
Tuesday	_____
Wednesday	_____
Thursday	_____
Friday	_____
Saturday	_____

Commitment Contract:

I, _____ will begin my new lifestyle on _____

at _____o'clock. I am committed to my new lifestyle, and I would like to achieve

my goal(s)of_____

_____

_____

_____

because _____

_____

_____

_____.

Signed_____ Date _____

Scouting Locations

Choosing locations for your workouts can be a lot of fun. Whether you live in town or out in the country, once you start looking at your environment as a place of opportunity for exercise, so many possibilities are revealed! Different environments all have locations and types of props that lend themselves to great workouts, and they also have their own particular challenges. If you live in the city, you'll naturally have a different set of factors—and potential hazards— to consider when working out than if you live in the mountains. Depending on where you live, and where you plan to take your outdoor workouts, consider these factors.

Urban Workouts

Look at your town or city with a fresh eye. You'll find surprising potential for your workouts.

Locations: Parks, plazas, playgrounds, stadiums, athletic fields, public walkways and paths, backyards.

TIP: Buy a map of your area. You'll be surprised by how many parks, pathways, and open areas have always been there—you just didn't know about them!

Props: Benches and tables. Curbs, concrete blocks, and walls. Steps, stairs, and bleachers. Mail boxes, stop signs, parking meters, and lamp posts. Grass, snow mounds, and sand pits. Playground apparatus and jungle gyms.

Environmental considerations:
- Traffic and cars
- Pedestrian traffic
- Air quality: pollution, exhaust, unsavory smells
- Potholes and cracked or uneven concrete streets and sidewalks
- Dogs—and dog debris

Rural Workouts

See your environment differently when you're looking for potential workout locations and props.

Locations: Parks, open fields, pastures, orchards and groves, hiking trails, dirt roads, school tracks, backyards.

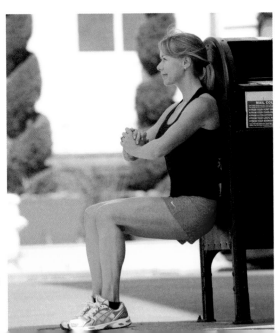

"Tree sits" can be done anywhere!

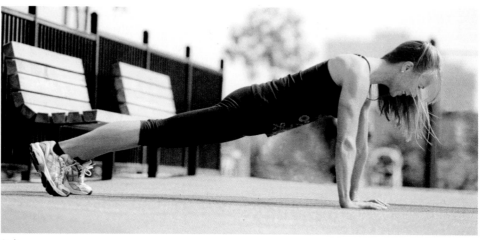

Push-up

Props: Trees, fallen logs, hillsides, creeks. Brick retention walls and steps cut into hillsides. Split fences. Grass, gravel, sand, snow, pine needles, leaves.

Environmental considerations:
- Risk of overexposure to elements, dust, animals, and insects
- Distance from emergency assistance
- Lack of cellular phone coverage

Beach and Shoreline Workouts

Everyday fixtures can give you a great workout.

Locations: Boardwalks and promenades, piers and docks, jetties, bicycle paths, sandy and rocky shorelines.

Props: Benches and picnic tables. Lifeguard stands. Sea walls. Docking

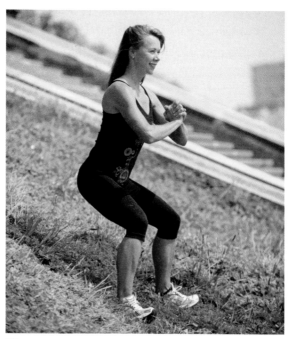

Hill squat

TIP: Try to scout your locations at the same hour of the day in which you plan to exercise there. You don't want to get caught midfield by the sprinkler system at 10 a.m.!

TIP: Find out what types of animals live in the area where you're working out, and learn the best steps to coexist with them safely.

cleats. Firm and soft sand. Sand dunes and shelves. Posts, poles, and fences. Driftwood and rocks.

Environmental considerations:

- Fishing debris (e.g., tackle and hooks) on piers or docks
- Tides and waves
- Broken glass and hidden debris in sand
- Sand can lead you to twist joints unintentionally

Mountain Workouts

The same path you've always followed offers new potential when you use a new perspective.

Locations: Hiking trails, fire roads, trails that follow and cut across streams. Dry riverbeds, lake shores, parks, and campgrounds. Forests and mountain meadows.

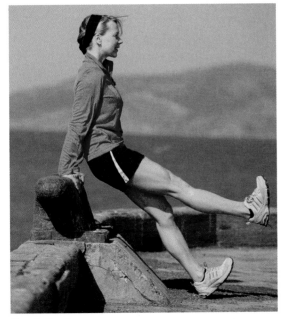

Use a docking cleat as a prop

Props: Boulders, trees, fallen trees, tree stumps, roots and branches. Sandy lake shores. Rock walls, fences, ledges. Pine-needle- and leaf-laden hillsides.

Environmental considerations:

- Altitude
- Prop safety, such as rotting logs and tree trunks
- Season/climate, such as sudden storms
- Animals and insects
- Sun exposure

TIP: A great test for air quality is the presence of lichen and moss. This family of algae and fungi, which grows on rocks, trees, and soil, from ocean shorelines to mountain peaks, will only grow where the air and other environmental conditions are clean.

Trail and Traffic Etiquette

When you exercise outdoors, you become part of a community that consists of the natural world around you and other people who are sharing the outdoor experience. Respect and attentiveness keep everyone safe, ensure a peaceful experience for all, and protect the natural environment. Here are some dos and don'ts for good behavior on the trail:

- Respect the quality of the outdoor experience. If you're working out in a pair or a group, observe quiet—don't chatter. If you do speak, use a low voice so the natural sound of nature will preside.
- Leave behind what you find. Enjoy the beauty of nature but skip the souvenirs. Leave plants, flowers, rocks, shells, and other objects as you found them.
- Help to maintain the trails. Carry a plastic bag to pick up small pieces of trash found along the way.
- Avoid being sideswiped. When merging onto a trail or across a path or road, always look to see if there is oncoming traffic.
- Call out your intentions. When approaching someone on a trail, you must announce your presence and your intentions. "Hi, I'm coming up behind you." "Passing on your left. Thank you."
- Pass others on the trail correctly. When passing on the trail, be sure to pass on the left or to the outside. If you're yielding to others, step to the right or the inside of the trail, away from the edge. When being passed on a trail with a drop-off on one side, step to the inside, against the hill.
- Admire wildlife from a distance. Never approach, feed, or touch animals.

Snot Rocket, Cannonball Blow, Air Hankie, Golfer's Blow

It's all about nose clearing on the fly. Experts call it exercise-induced rhinorrhea, and it's common in athletes and a fact of life for many outdoor-exercise enthusiasts. I call it flying biohazards! As a coach, trainer, and the best friend of one offender, I've been sprayed and spit on, and I've taken it upon myself to be the "habit breaker" for many. No matter what you call it, it's rude and can be dangerous for fellow exercisers in your path, potentially spreading illness or disease. So carry a tissue, and be discreet and aware of who is around.

• Stay on marked trails. Do not create new trails or erode existing ones.

Choosing Your Workout

Another factor in choosing your location is the type of workout you're planning. Each of Outdoor Fitness's three types of workouts—single site, multisite, and traveling—have characteristics that lend themselves to particular locations.

Single-Site Workouts

Single-site workouts are sessions that take place entirely in one spot. These workouts are convenient and efficient, perfect for days when you're pressed for time or when you want to focus on muscular strength and endurance. Parks, playgrounds, backyards, steps or stairs, and hillsides are all good locations for single-site workouts. Some single-site workouts are best executed on flat ground, and others adapt well to uneven terrain. To keep things interesting, think about choosing places—and times of day—that will provide lots of great visual stimulation to keep your mind engaged: the colors and textures of a park on a fall day, the beauty of a hillside at sunset, the city waking up on an early morning along the waterfront.

Multisite Workouts

Multisite workouts are great for large parks, stadiums, long stretches of beach or shoreline, or a mountain trail loop. Full of cardiovascular and muscular conditioning, multisite workouts offer flexibility and versatility. You choose a route and stop for exercises along the way, creating stations for your strength training mixed with blocks of cardio that transport you to from station to station. Your local schools have athletic fields with bleachers and tracks perfect for multisite sessions. Find a path that winds around a pond, or create an out-and-back session along a river way. Use your imagination!

Traveling Workouts

Traveling workouts are full of adventure. In these workouts, you'll plan to cover anywhere from 1 to 5 miles. You have so many choices with traveling workouts: You can take a long cardio session out to a site where you'll perform your strength training exercises, or you can intersperse your exercises along the route. Some of the most scenic locations are also the best ones for traveling locations: large parks, lakeside paths, mountain trails. You'll be working across different types of terrain, so it's especially important to pay attention to the changes along your route.

TIP: The number-one piece of equipment is a pair of well fitting shoes made for the activity and terrain you'll be working with.

Gearing Up

So what do you need for an Outdoor Fitness workout? Very little! One of the greatest perks of Outdoor Fitness is that it doesn't require extensive equipment. All that is truly necessary is a well-fitting, functional pair of shoes. Having the right footwear for the terrain is vital. Wearing the wrong shoes for the activity is like driving a Formula One racecar on a bumpy mountain fire road. There are two main types of shoes that are best suited to Outdoor Fitness workouts:

All-terrain shoes are great for rural environments and off-road running. This type of shoe supports climbing, descending, and traversing uneven ground and will help you hold onto wet rocks and roots. Shoes made with Gore-Tex material are helpful in wet conditions.

Shoes for walking and running on the road work well in an urban environment. Their firm construction protects your feet on pavement and concrete. Choose the shoe that best suits the environment where you'll be working out.

Regardless of the shoe you select, a good fit is essential. Squeezing into a shoe that is too small can cause pinched

Tips for Buying and Caring for Your Shoes

- Shop after a workout or at the end of the day, when your feet have swelled from activity.
- Take a quick jog around the block before you buy the shoes.
- Take your worn-out shoes with you when shopping for new ones. They hold clues to any special conditions you might have.
- To make shoes last, buy two pairs and rotate them.
- Follow the 25 percent rule. If you engage in an activity like running more than 25 percent of the week, add a shoe made specifically for that activity.
- Never wash your shoes in hot water. Use cold water, on the gentle cycle, and air dry them.
- Replace your shoes every three to five months, depending on use.

nerves, bunions, hammertoes, corns, and blisters. Shoes that are too large can cause accidents—a loose fit leads to a lack of control.

Don't take shortcuts with your footwear. Foot problems eventually spread to other areas of the body, including ankles, knees, hips, and lower back.

Safety First

Let common sense be your guide when choosing both locations and props. Always ask yourself: Is this a safe spot for the work I want to do? Scan your environment for dips in the ground, potholes, and loose rocks. Make sure you test out your props for stability before performing your exercises. Benches should be stable and well constructed, tree trunks healthy and sturdy, boulders well planted and secure in the ground, before you put your full weight on them in an exercise.

Adapting to the Elements

Outdoor Fitness is an all-season, all-climate workout program. Changing seasons offer new stimulation for your body, your mind, and your senses. The variety and fluctuation of the weather and seasonal changes keep you chal-

lenged, enhancing the pleasure of exercising outdoors.

We have a saying at Outdoor Fitness: There's no such thing as inappropriate weather, only inappropriate clothing. Since 1995, I've cancelled only two classes because of weather—one due to high winds and the other due to lightning. Outdoor Fitness is made for all seasons. However, all types of weather pose challenges and often hazards. In seasons that include severe weather—hot or cold temperatures, or high altitude—you'll need to put your body through a period of adjustment, or acclimation, as you gradually grow accustomed to the conditions.

The key to staying safe and having fun exercising outdoors year-round is to be aware of the obstacles and potential hazards that the elements pose—and to prepare yourself to avoid them. Rain, wind, snow, heat, and cold: Outdoor Fitness has strategies for you to work out safely and comfortably no matter what the forecast.

Heat

Many people love the feeling of working out in hot weather. The sun, the sweat, and the gorgeous scenery all make outdoor workouts appealing in the summertime. There is plenty of fun to be had in the sun, provided you're aware of the

> ### How Hot is Too Hot? Temperature Guidelines for Hot-Weather Workouts
>
> **80°F and below:** Low risk. If properly hydrated and acclimated, there is slim chance of heat-related illness.
>
> **81°F–87°F:** Moderate risk. Stay hydrated, seek shade, and avoid heavy exertion. Remember that the risk rises with the humidity level.
>
> **88°F and above:** High risk. Exercise only if you are acclimated for the heat and humidity. Work out earlier in the day, and drink plenty of fluids.

risks. Heat is the most dangerous element you face in exercising outdoors. As the temperature rises, your body must work harder to keep your core temperature cool. This causes your system to use up fluids quickly. Hydrate! Hydrate! Hydrate! This is your mantra during hot-weather exercise.

To exercise safely in hot weather, follow these guidelines:

- **Hydrate.** Before and after a workout, drink 8 to 10 ounces of water. For workouts longer than 50 to 60 minutes, carry water with you.
- **Dress to let your skin breathe.** Wear reflective light-or white-colored, nonconstrictive, breathable fabrics to maximize sweat evaporation. Cottons and silks work, as do many synthetics and blends. Avoid nonbreathable or rubberized garments.
- **Protect your skin.** Use sweatproof sunscreen with SPF 15 or higher.
- **Wear sunglasses.** Always wear lightweight UVA- and UVB-protected eyewear.
- **Protect your head.** A sun visor or cap in bright or light sun-reflective colors will shield your face and eyes.
- **Get out early.** Exercise in the early morning before the intensity of the day's heat. Even if it feels cooler at the end of the day, the ground will give off absorbed heat for hours.
- **Go gradually.** Acclimate gradually by exercising before 10:00 a.m. for 15 minutes. Build up to 60 minutes over three to four weeks.

Hot weather combined with high humidity poses particular risks for heat stress and heat stroke, and extra precautions are necessary to avoid illness and injury. Be cautious when temperatures rise above 76 degrees Fahrenheit and 75 percent humidity. If you are working out in hot, humid weather, pay even more attention to hydration, making sure you drink cold water before, during, and after your workouts. Know the warning signs for heat injuries, such as heat stress, heat stroke, and sunstroke:

- Muscle cramps
- Skin rash
- Lethargy
- Irritability
- Elevated heart rate
- Headache
- Dizziness
- Nausea and vomiting
- Hot, flushed, and dry skin
- Lack of perspiration
- An altered state of consciousness, confusion, or poor judgment

Cold

Winter can be an exhilarating time to exercise outdoors. Snow-capped mountains, glistening hillsides, and crisp cool air are enticing. Winter weather often drives people into the gym, so you're likely to have the trail to yourself. Cold

Keys to Winter Safety

- Wear suitable clothing.
- Wear all-terrain running or light hiking shoes.
- Limit your time outdoors if you're not conditioned for the cold—don't stay out all day.
- Have a change of clothes for after your workout.
- Have access to a shelter.
- Choose alternative routes if your regular route seems risky. Consider shorter loops, rather than traveling far from your starting point.
- Wear brightly colored clothing to be visible to drivers.
- Use caution on snow-covered surfaces, which may be hiding obstacles—such as pinecones and rocks—underneath.
- Carry a cell phone.

temperatures, snow, and ice all pose risks you need to prepare for.

Maintaining your body heat is the first priority in cold-weather exercise. If you keep a healthy core temperature, the cold around you will have little effect on either your health or your performance. A drop in core temperature can lead to hypothermia, which is when your body begins to generate heat by excessive muscular oscillation.

Hypothermia is marked by these symptoms:

- Shivering
- Feeling cold to the core, with goose bumps and numbing
- Loss of coordination and sluggishness
- Difficulty speaking, mental confusion, and stumbling
- Unconsciousness

Dressing appropriately is the best defense against a drop in your body

TIP: Perhaps the most hazardous part of a cold-weather workout is after the workout, when your body is cooling down. Problems with chilling can arise due to wet skin from perspiration, because the blood vessels in the skin continue to dilate to dissipate heat. It is potentially dangerous because this is when the body feels warm, so most people don't feel the need to bundle up. If you are not heading home right away, always have a change of clothing available. The effects of chilling from wet clothing and wet skin come on rapidly and are difficult to abate without a hot shower or bath.

temperature and is the ticket to a great workout in chilly weather. Cold-weather dressing is all about layers and fabrics. Avoid wearing cotton, which loses up to 80 percent of its insulating capabilities when it's wet. Cotton clothes can actually contribute to hypothermia. Technical fabrics (synthetic fabrics and clothing designed to easily adjust to your body temperature) are created specifically to function in cold temperatures. Follow these guidelines for maintaining your core temperature and protecting your body in cold weather:

- **Layer clothing.** Several thin layers work better than one heavy layer. Layers are also easier to add or remove to regulate temperature. The goal is to keep warm, minimize sweating, and avoid shivering.
- **Cover your head.** Up to 50 percent of body heat can be lost through your head. Always wear a hat or a headband.
- **Wear gloves.** To insulate and protect your hands, choose lightweight gloves that provide the greatest warmth and flexibility, preferably with rubberized or leather strips on the palm for gripping props.
- **Cover your mouth.** A scarf or mask will help to warm the air before you breathe it. This is especially important if you have respiratory problems, such

as asthma, which can be irritated by cold air.

- **Stay dry.** Wet, damp clothing—from either perspiration or precipitation—significantly increases heat loss.
- **Keep your feet dry.** Choose socks made of polypropylene, wool, or another fabric that wicks moisture and retains insulation when the feet get wet.
- **Wear sunglasses.** Select lightweight shields with UVA and UVB protection. Some styles have interchangeable lenses for sunlight, flat light, and foggy conditions.
- **Stay hydrated.** Dehydration affects the body's ability to regulate heat. Fluids—especially water—are as important in cold weather as in hot weather. Avoid alcohol and caffeine, which dehydrate your system and constrict your blood vessels.

Cold-Weather Fabrics

For cold weather, you want to go technical all the way. Cold-weather clothing can be classified according to function and layering categories:

Base layer: the first layer next to skin. Choose a lightweight technical fabric that breathes, wicks away perspiration, keeps your body insulated, and allows freedom of movement.

Middle layer: absorbs moisture and provides insulation. Depending on the temperature, choose pants or leggings for the lower half, and on top, choose a long-sleeved, zip-neck jersey. Or if it's really chilly, choose a nonpilling fleece fabric for this layer, like microfleece.

Outer layer or shell layer: protects from the elements. You'll want a quality garment for protection from wind, rain, and snow, so again, go technical. Whether the weather warrants a lightweight waterproof shell or blizzardproof shell, select garments that have been seam sealed and allow body heat to evaporate while shielding your skin from the elements.

Altitude

No matter what your fitness level, significant changes in altitude pose challenges for your body because of the reduced oxygen in the air. Traveling above 5,000 to 6,000 feet can have immediate effects on our bodies. If you take your training to an altitude that you are not used to—for example, if you routinely exercise at sea level and travel to an elevation of 8,000 feet—you'll need to decrease the intensity of your sessions to allow your body to adapt.

Skipping this acclimation process can bring about adverse reactions associated with altitude sickness, such as headache, nausea, fatigue, and sleeplessness, as well as cerebral and pulmonary edema. As a general guideline, you'll need two weeks to adapt to altitudes up to 7,500 feet, adding an additional week for every 2,000-foot increase.

Rain

There's no reason to halt your workout because of rain. In the event of a showery, wet day, you'll need to take some extra precautions. Consider the effect of the rain on the route you've planned and make a change if you think the conditions will be too slippery. (Even in warm weather, rain can make a surface slick.) Pay extra attention to wet leaves, twigs, and rocks on the path.

TIP: Time and time again, I've seen clients begin their session a little intimidated by the rain. But after the warm-up, they've forgotten it's raining, and by the cooldown all I see are smiles. The sense of accomplishment is overwhelming, the feeling is invigorating, and the outcome is right on track! I liken workouts in the rain to jumping into a swimming pool. The first couple of minutes take some getting used to. The rest—you forget you're wet!

Wind

You might not give a second thought to the effects of wind on your workout, but windy conditions can bring about many changes and new obstacles to your route. Be sure to wear sunglasses or other protective eyewear since blowing dust, dirt, and sand can spoil a session. Watch closely for debris on your path, from small twigs to branches and pinecones. Dress to protect yourself against the wind—wind chill accelerates cooling, so make sure to add layers if it's already cool outside. Familiarize yourself with a wind barrier—a large tree or a wall—to use as a shield if the wind conditions become severe.

Pesky Bugs and Poisonous Plants

Neither poisonous plants nor annoying bugs should be a deterrent to exercising outdoors. Familiarizing yourself with the insects and plants in your region, in order to avoid contact, is the best way to keep from having your outdoor workout ruined.

Quick Facts about Poisonous Plants

- Poisonous plants grow in all U.S. states, with the exception of Hawaii and Alaska.
- Poison oak is common to the Ameri-

can West and Southeast, as well as Canada.

- Poison ivy and poison sumac are found in the American East and southern Canada.
- More than half of humans are allergic to poison oak, ivy, and sumac. Contact with these plants is the number-one cause of allergic skin reactions in the United States.

How to Prevent Insect Bites and Stings

- Wear light clothing. Dress in long-sleeved shirts and long pants.
- Avoid wearing perfume.
- Do not set up workouts near ripe fruit trees or sweet-smelling flowers.
- Stay on well-worn paths when you're in tick-infested areas such as thick forests, dense brush, or high grass.
- Shower immediately after you've returned from outdoor activity. Before showering, inspect your skin for ticks, especially under armpits, behind the knees, and around the groin.
- The best insect repellents contain DEET.

How to Avoid Snakes

- Know if there are venomous snakes in the area.
- Use caution around boulders, rock piles, wood piles, tree roots, thick leaves and brush, and tall grass.
- Never step over a fallen tree or large rock. Step onto it to see if there is a snake tucked into the other side.
- Don't dig around in dark places—such as hollow logs, trees, or holes—with your bare hands.
- If you see a snake, leave it alone. Snakes aren't aggressive, though they will strike to defend themselves. If the snake doesn't leave, calmly back away.
- Never poke or prod a snake with a stick.

Injuries, Aches, and Pains

In Outdoor Fitness, most injuries can be avoided altogether by wearing proper clothes and shoes, by giving your body a full warm-up and cooldown, and by sticking to a gradual and progressive training program. Your most important tool for preventing injury is your concentration: Moment-to-moment focus on the task at hand is the surest way to stay safe and injury-free throughout even your most challenging workouts.

Exercise and athletics inevitably bring about aches, muscle fatigue, and soreness. These are part of the territory for active people. Ignoring your aches

TIP: The number-one cause of injuries with Outdoor Fitness is a lapse in mental focus.

and pains is a mistake. Left unattended, mild pain, fatigue, and soreness can develop into something more serious and debilitating. It's important to listen to your body and to avoid overtraining so that those aches and pains do not develop into full-blown injuries.

Too Far Too Fast— Overtraining and Injury

Overtraining is the most common cause of injury and physical ailments. In a rush to accomplish too much too soon, people often do themselves—and their fitness goals—real harm. Play it smart, and you'll stay healthy, make steady progress, and enjoy your exercise uninterrupted by injury and fatigue. Overdo things, and you'll risk a host of injuries, including shin splints, stress fractures, ankle sprains, knee and lower-back pain, and foot pain. Know the signs of pushing yourself too hard, and learn how to pull back and give your body the rest it needs. Use pain as your general guide. If something hurts, stop doing it. Your body is remarkably adept at sensing the seriousness of an injury and responding accordingly. Resist the temptation to

Symptoms of Overtraining

- An unusual feeling of tiredness and fatigue
- An early-morning resting pulse with an increase of five or more beats
- Muscles that may be unusually sore
- Loss of appetite and weight loss
- Cold or viral infections
- Emotional distress—anxiety, tension, anger, or depression
- A lack of interest in training
- Difficulty focusing or making decisions
- Bowel changes—diarrhea or constipation

stretch an injured muscle—this can often make things worse, as you risk tearing muscle fibers.

Accidents on the Trail

Injuries from overuse can happen gradually, and it's rare to have an injury occur in the middle of a workout; however, you need to be prepared. Soft tissue injuries such as sprains, pulls, and bruises should be tended to immediately.

If you do experience an injury during your workout, ask yourself the following questions to determine if it is serious:

- Is there pain? Dull or sharp?
- Is there redness or swelling?
- Is the injured side different from the other side?
- Is there warmth? This could be a sign of inflammation.
- Can you move it? If not, can you stand on it or move it through its range of motion?

If an injury has been identified, or if you are not really sure, stop the activity immediately and seek medical assistance. You can also try the RICER method: rest, ice, compression, elevation, referral. RICER is also an appropriate treatment for many injuries brought about by overuse. If you're unsure about how to treat your injury, don't try to go it alone. Ask your doctor's advice.

The RICER method is broken down as follows:

R—Rest: Slows down any bleeding and reduces the risk of further damage.

I—Ice: Eases pain, reduces initial bleeding, and later encourages blood flow.

C—Compression: Reduces bleeding and swelling.

E—Elevation: Reduces bleeding and swelling by allowing fluids to flow away from the injury.

R—Referral: If you're concerned about severe injury, or if pain and swelling do not improve over 48 hours, seek medical help.

In the first 24 hours after an injury, you should avoid applying heat to the affected area. Heat causes swelling and further inflammation. This includes

Applying Ice

- Ice must never be applied directly to the skin. If you don't have a cloth-covered ice pack, wrap your ice pack in a towel or T-shirt to prevent burns.

- Apply ice for about 20 minutes to control internal bleeding and swelling. Continue to ice in this way every 2 hours for the next 48 hours. This will vary depending on the size of the area and the depth of the damaged tissue. Icing can be reduced gradually over the next 24 to 48 hours.

showers, baths, and saunas. Don't drink alcohol, either: Drinking can mask the pain and severity of an injury, as well as increase bleeding and swelling. Avoid deep tissue massage for at least 72 hours after injury. And don't skimp on your rest: 72 hours is a general rule for returning to exercise after injury, unless you've received the okay from your doctor to resume activity sooner.

You're now ready to get going. Get your shoes on, pull out those sunglasses, and lather up with sunscreen. It's time to get outdoors and start working out in a whole new way!

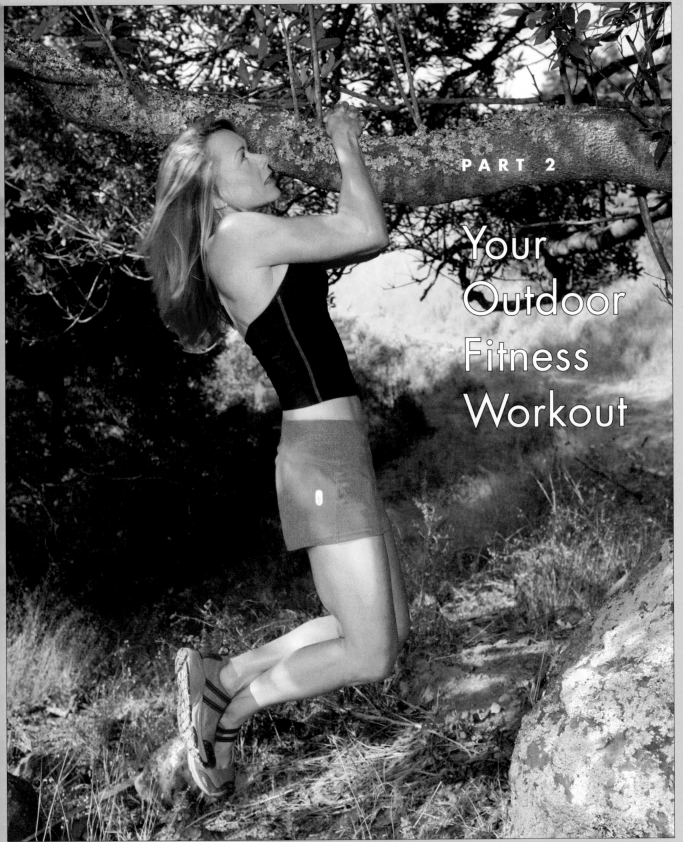

PART 2

Your
Outdoor
Fitness
Workout

MITCHEL SHENKER

CHAPTER 4

How to Begin and End an Outdoor Fitness Workout: Warm Up and Cool Down

Before you get started with your new Outdoor Fitness program, I want to give you an overview of the exercises and moves that you will be doing when you warm up and cool down before and after each workout. The warm-up and cooldown are important parts of the Outdoor Fitness workout, which is made up of several different components:

1. **The warm-up:** Warms your muscles and joints and gets your heart moving.

2. **Form and alignment:** This teaches you proper posture and body alignment so you can maximize the effecta of an exercise without injuring yourself.

3. **Strengthening exercises and endurance training:** These focus on strengthening your muscles, joints, and skeleton, using Base Moves, which are the exercises that form the foundation of any Outdoor Fitness workout (you'll learn these in Phase 1, found in chapter 5), and Signature Moves, which continue to develop your skills and your strength, focusing more on your core (your abdominals and torso), your arms, and your back. (You'll learn these in Phase 2, found in chapter 6.)

4. **Cooldown and flexibility:** During the cooldown you not only bring your heart rate to a resting state, but you also take time to stretch your muscles. Please note that you can use these stretches after—or during—your warm-up and before you do any strengthening exercises.

The Warm-Up

Every workout begins with a 5- to 10-minute warm-up. A warm-up is your time to limber up your body—and your mind—in preparation for the workout to come. It can be as simple as a walk or a jog. My warm-ups combine breathing and posture exercises with joint lubrication exercises, followed by an environmental integration exercise I call "high toes." I've also included a couple of "one-spot warm-up" exercises that are perfect for situations when you aren't including a walk to your workout site as part of your warm-up.

Joint Lubrication

Starting with your lower body and moving upward, this series of gentle exercises will loosen your joints, releasing stiffness and tension. Standing on one leg, extend the other leg forward and circle your ankle to the right and then to the left. Take your time and use your full range of motion. Repeat the rotations twice more in each direction. Continue, moving upward to your knees, hips, wrists, elbows, and shoulders, move each joint through its range of motion three times. Now move on to the other leg.

Ankle rotation

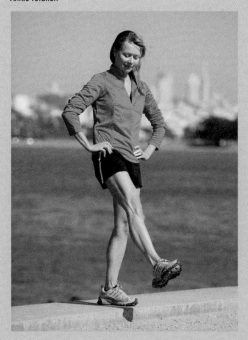 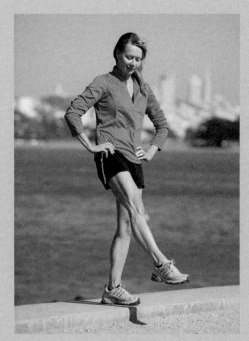

Knee extension

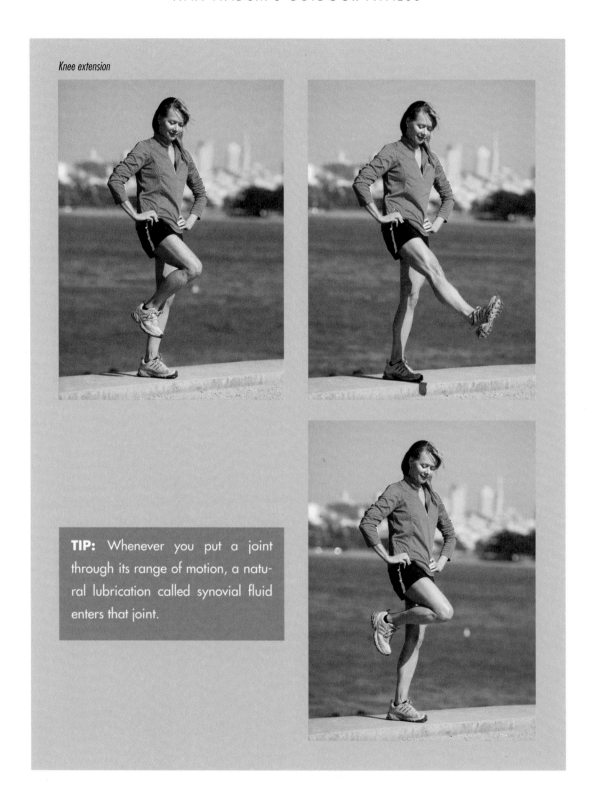

TIP: Whenever you put a joint through its range of motion, a natural lubrication called synovial fluid enters that joint.

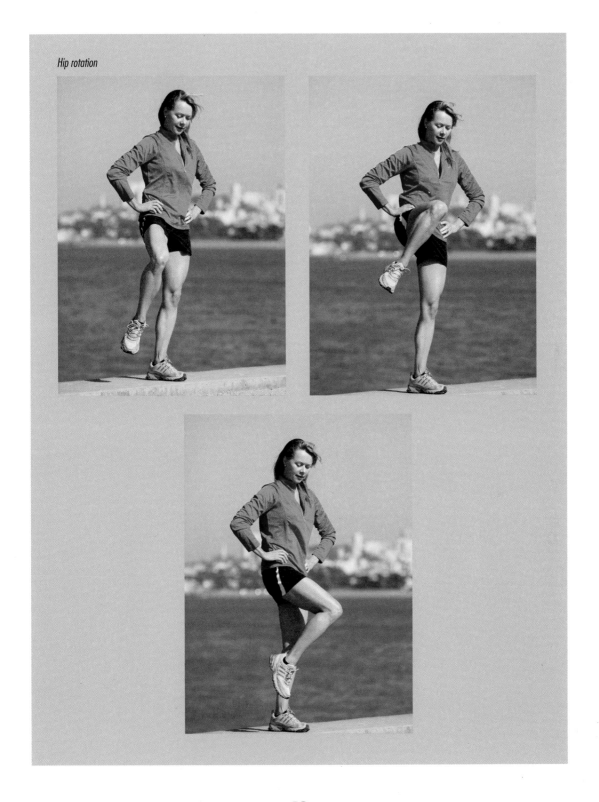

Hip rotation

Wrist rotation

Elbow flexing

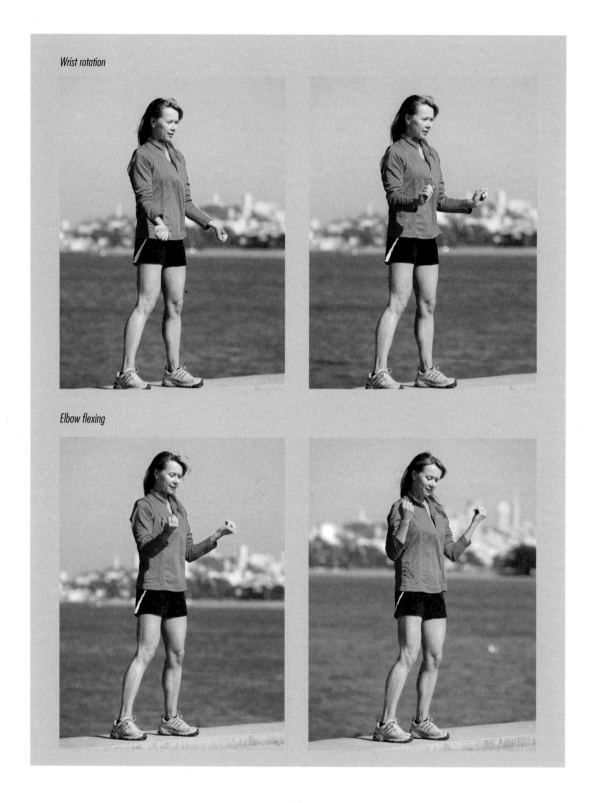

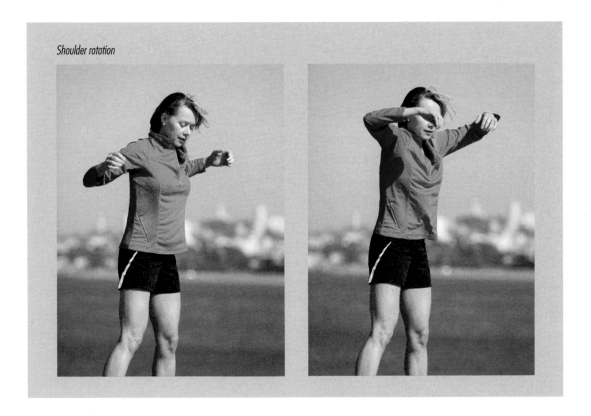

Shoulder rotation

Reverse Breath

Position yourself in the athletic stance (see Get into Proper Starting Position in chapter 5). Take a deep breath: an easy inhale followed by a slow exhale. Empty your lungs of air as you exhale completely—all the way out. When you next breathe in, observe how your lungs expand to accommodate the air that rushes in to replenish the breath you've exhaled. Repeat with a second breath.

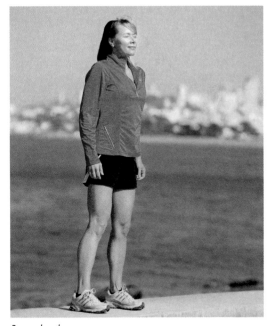

Reverse breath

Posture Check

Stand tall, eyes forward, chin up, and ribs lifted up and away from your pelvis. Take in a deep breath as you rotate your shoulders up and back. Exhale as you bring your shoulders down, away from your ears, drawing your shoulder blades together. Feel your chest open as you take a couple more breaths. Allow your arms to hang loosely at your sides. Observe the change in your posture.

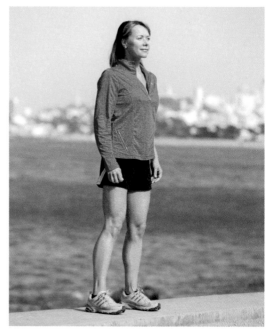

Posture check

Cardio Warm-Up (and Cooldown)

A cardio warm-up is often part of the general warm-up, which helps you get your heart rate up and gives you time to get to know the terrain around you—especially what you'll encounter underfoot. For example, you might begin with a fast walk using your high toes technique (see below), creating awareness of everything in your path. Feel for those stray pebbles, twigs, and cracks in the sidewalk, the dips and bumps in the road. Are you clearing rocks and roots that pop up on the trail smoothly and without tripping?

As you become more comfortable with the terrain, you may want to bump up your speed by pumping your arms to set the tempo of your feet. After a couple of minutes, you should be at a Rate of Perceived Exertion (RPE) of 4 to 5. Keep bumping up your pace gradually until you reach an RPE of 6 to 7, and continue for a few more minutes. As you reach your destination, you'll want to walk it out for 30 seconds or so, bringing your RPE down to a 5 or 6. Now stretch or move into your workout.

At the end of your workout, I often suggest a cardio cooldown to gradually bring your heart rate down before you do your stretching. Examples of this would be a slow jog or a fast walk.

Heel-Toe Roll and High Toes

Two techniques that I teach my clients right away are the heel-toe roll and high toes. When you use a heel-toe roll, you hit the ground heel first, roll through your foot to your toes, and use your toes to propel you forward. A great way to get the feeling for this is to imagine your feet to be like tires of a car, rolling over the terrain.

With high toes, you keep your toes up as your feet skim the ground to prevent tripping over obstacles in your path. Imagine that there is air running between your feet and the ground, and you are just floating above the terrain.

Both these techniques help build kinesthetic and proprioceptive awareness in your feet—and enable you to feel through your feet. (See page 62 for RPE suggestions.)

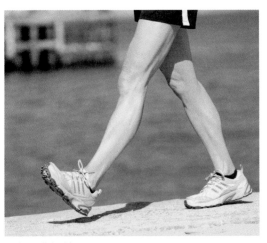

Heel-toe roll, heel first

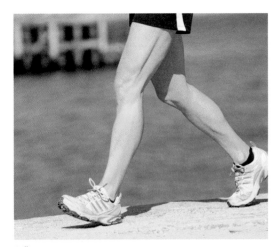

Roll to your toes

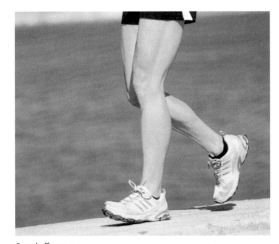

Propel off your toes

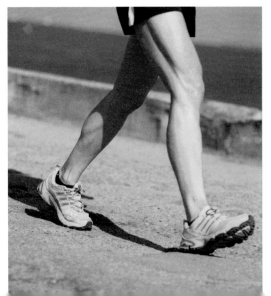

High toes

Flexibility

While technically you don't have to stretch during your warm-up session, I usually recommend that you include the "four basics"—hip flexors, hamstrings, quadriceps, and calves. If lunges are part of your workout, include the adductors (inner thigh) as your fifth stretch. (See the Cooldown and Flexibility section of this chapter for descriptions of these.)

High Knees

Next, let's loosen your hips and engage your core with high knees. This warm-up exercise will also get your heart pumping a little faster and ready to move into your workout.

- Take an athletic stance and set your posture: Engage your center of mass by lifting your ribs up and away from your hips, chest open, eyes forward, and chin up. Keep your arms extended in front of you between chest and navel height.

- Begin by marching in place. Lift your knees up and away in front of your body, making contact with your hands and creating a reverse curl in the lower abdominal wall. Keep your hips even and square with your shoulders as you march. Feel your abdominal wall begin to engage. Extend height. Keep your ribs lifted as you continue to lift and lower your knees up to your hands, palms down, bringing your knees up to touch your palms.

- After about 20 to 30 seconds, begin to lift your knees more diagonally and out toward the sides for a count of 10. After 10, gradually bring your knees back to center and your original position. As you become stronger and more flexible, you can lift both your hands and your knees higher.

High knees

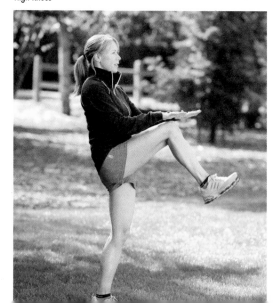
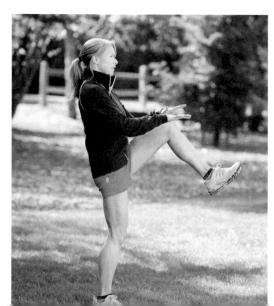

"One-Spot Warm-up"

Use a "one-spot warm-up" for those times when you aren't able to walk or jog for a warm-up. Use a step, curb, or berm for step-ups, kickbacks, and lateral lifts. After 5 to 8 minutes, walk it out, and then move on to flexibility, high knees, and your workout.

Step-Ups with a Kickback

Step up with your left foot, making full foot contact—especially through the heel—as you rise up. Lift your right foot behind you as you contract your glutes. Then place your right foot back on the ground, followed by your left foot back to the ground. Alternate lead legs and create a rhythm: "Up, kickback, down, down . . . Up, kickback, down, down." As you march, think about maintaining great posture and stepping down softly through the ball of your foot.

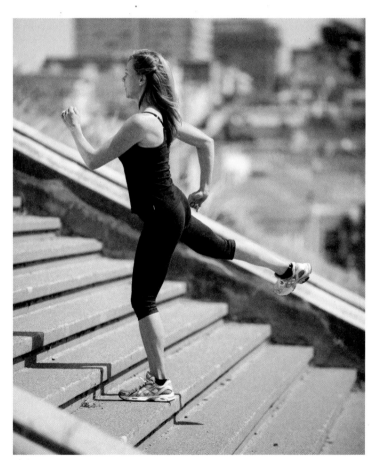

Kickbacks are great for a one-spot warm-up

Lateral Lifts

Next, stand laterally to the step, with your hands on your hips. Use your right foot to step sideways onto the step, and lift your left leg out to the side. Step down onto your left foot. Follow with the right foot and tap the ground before stepping up again and repeating the leg lift. Pay close attention to your form and posture. Are your hips squared, and are your ribs lifted? Is your chin up? Are you breathing deeply? At the 30-second mark, switch legs. Step with your left foot and lift your right leg for another 30 seconds.

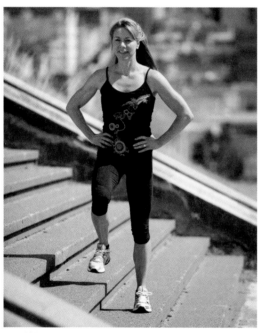

Lateral lifts — step up

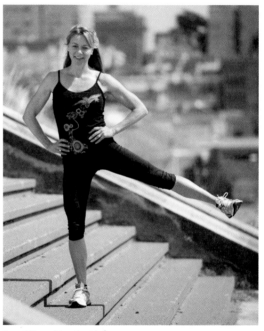

Lateral lifts — lift to the side

Cooldown and Flexibility

End your workout with gentle, stimulating, and soothing stretches that will clear your mind and relax your limbs. As you wind down, breathe, feel your body, and continue to integrate your being with the environment around you. *Note:* You can use props, like a step, log, rock, or curb, for the stretches that follow.

The cooldown phase of your workout is as important as the warm-up. By taking the time to cool down properly, you allow your body to unwind from its exertion, prevent stiffness and pain, and give yourself time to clear your mind before resuming your busy day.

Here is an example of an effective cooldown:

Cardio Cooldown (RPE 5)

When you are at the tail end of your workout and heading back to your starting point, hold your pace at an RPE of 5. Use your low and slow breathing to wash your body with oxygen and clear out any lactic acid. Also, use this segment to clear your body and your mind of any tension.

PMJ Technique

Maximize your time and prepare for the rest of your day with a moving meditation. You've already learned that most of our thoughts can be broken down into three types: plans, memories, and judgments. Now try using this mindfulness exercise out on the path to clear your mind, root out the cobwebs, and let go of any lingering tension or stress:

As you walk or jog back to your starting point, center yourself with a few deep breaths. Connect to this moment through your breath, paying attention to your body moving and the terrain underfoot. Keep your mind clear while still noticing the colors, textures, and smells around you. If a thought should arise, quickly identify it and release it. Is it a plan? A memory? A judgment? Notice that once the thought is identified, it is released. Poof. Gone. Like magic, your mind is clear again. Continue to bring your mind back to the present moment. Walk it out, and move on to your cooldown flexibility stretches.

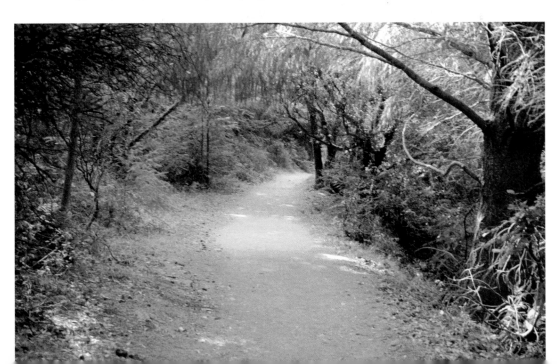

Flexibility Moves

Here are some basic rules when it comes to stretching:

- Never stretch a cold muscle.
- Warm up for 5 to 10 minutes before stretching (longer on chilly days).
- Hold a stretch for 20 to 30 seconds, for a total of about three breaths.
- Inhale to prepare for a stretch, and exhale while lengthening the muscles.
- Take the time to align and balance yourself on uneven ground.
- Don't bounce—it can cause injury to muscles, tendons, and ligaments.
- Pay attention to pain. If it hurts, stop the stretch.

Hip Flexor Stretch

Standing with your feet shoulder-width apart, take a giant step forward with your right foot into a lunge position. Align your front knee directly over your front heel. With your arms hanging loosely at your sides, slowly bend your knees until your fingertips touch the ground; at this point your left knee is resting on the ground and your left toes are pointed down. Take a deep breath in, and as you exhale, allow your hips to sink into the stretch. Repeat with your right leg.

MODIFICATION

Hip flexor stretch with a prop. Follow the same instructions as above, only place the center of your foot along the edge of a bench, block, stump, or log.

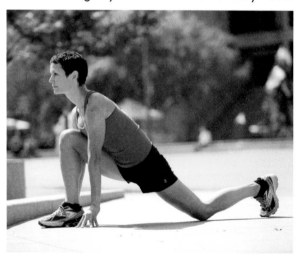

Hip flexor stretch

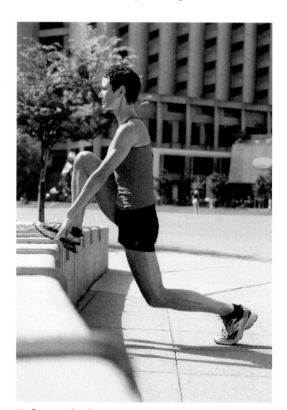

Hip flexor stretch with prop

Hamstring Stretch

Standing with your feet shoulder-width apart, step forward about 6 to 8 inches with your right foot. Flex your right foot so that the heel is on the ground and the toes are pointing up. Bend your knees slightly, place your hands on your thighs, and press your buttocks backward while keeping your back straight. As you begin to feel the stretch along the back of your right leg, tilt your tailbone up toward the sky. Hold. Repeat with your left leg.

MODIFICATION

Hamstring stretch with a prop. Follow the same instructions as above, but place your right heel on a curb, step, or log for leverage.

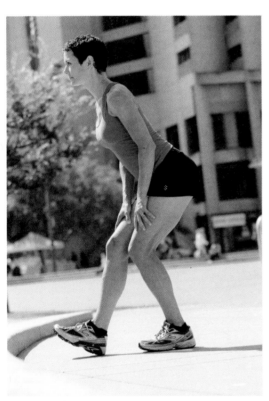

Hamstring stretch

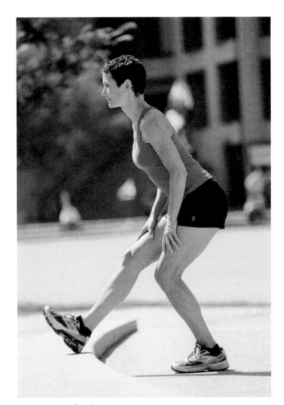

Hamstring stretch with prop

Quadriceps

Ground your feet on a firm surface and find a focal point. Place all your weight on your right leg. Bend your left leg behind you and grasp your instep with your left hand. With your left knee slightly behind your right leg, press your left hip forward while keeping your back straight and abs tight, and hold. You can lift your right arm perpendicular to the ground for added balance. Repeat with the right leg.

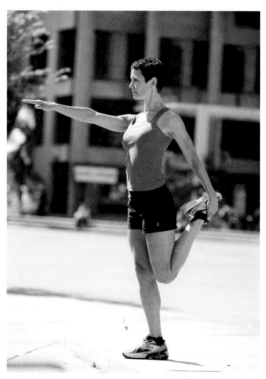

Quadriceps stretch

Calves

Stand facing a wall, tree, or post, approximately 1 foot away, with your feet together. Place your right heel as close to the prop as is comfortable, with the ball of your foot pressing against it, forming a 45-degree angle (keep your left foot on the ground). Gently push your right heel into the ground as you slowly roll up on the ball of your left foot and lean your upper body into the prop. Hold the stretch. Repeat with your left leg.

MODIFICATION

Alternative calf stretch. Hang one heel over the edge of a curb or step and feel the lengthening of your calf muscles. Repeat with the other leg.

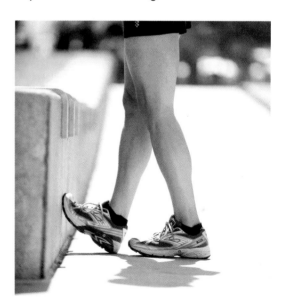

Calf stretch with prop

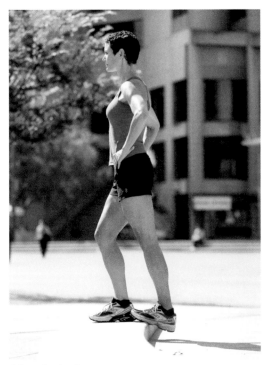

Calf stretch with curb

Inner Thighs (Adductors)

From the athletic stance, extend your right leg laterally, resting on your right heel, with your toes up in a diagonal position. Slowly, bend the left knee, keeping the knee over the heel, until you feel a light stretch in your inner thigh (right adductor). Hold the stretch. Repeat with the left leg.

MODIFICATION

Inner thigh (adductor) stretch with a prop. Follow the same instructions as above, but place your right heel on a curb, step, or log for leverage.

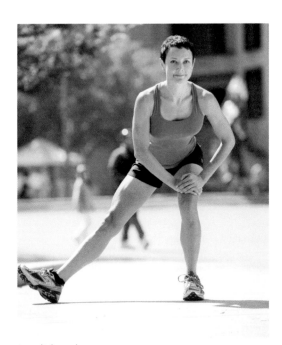

Inner thigh stretch

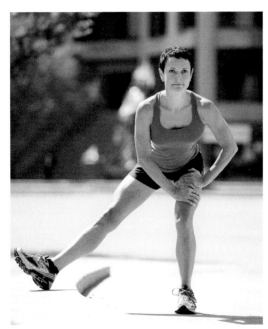

Inner thigh stretch with prop

Chest, Shoulders, Biceps

Clasp your hands together behind your back. As you press your chest forward, lift your arms up and away from your body. Feel a gentle stretch across your chest, shoulders, and biceps.

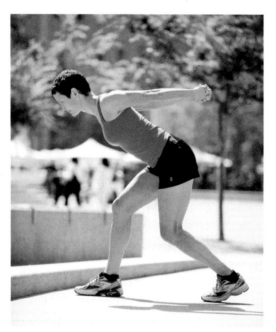

Chest/shoulder/bicep stretch

Back

Using a tree or post for assistance, face the object and lace your fingers together around it. Step back into a split stance, drawing back through the hips and pressing in to stretch the area between the shoulder blades.

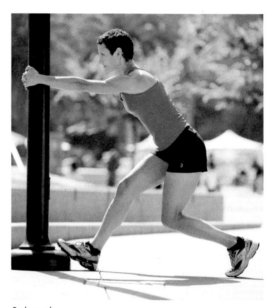

Back stretch

Upper Back and Rear Shoulders

Draw your straight right arm across your upper chest. Place your left hand on the back side of the upper right arm and press it into your body to release the muscles. Repeat on the left side.

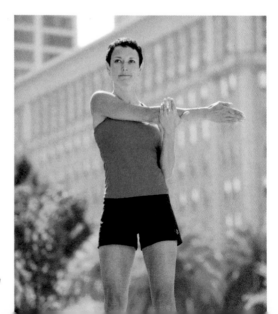

Upper back/shoulder stretch

Triceps

Lift your right arm up to the sky. Bend your arm at the elbow and reach your fingertips down your spine. Place the palm of your left hand on top of your right elbow and apply gentle pressure to assist release of the muscles.

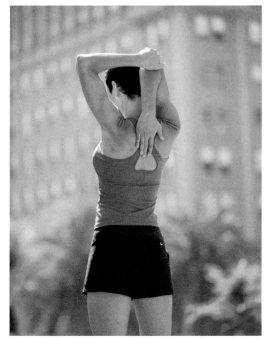

Triceps stretch

Torso

Stretch out your torso by reaching above your head with your right hand, then alternating with your left. Manipulate the stretch so that you feel it down the length of your torso.

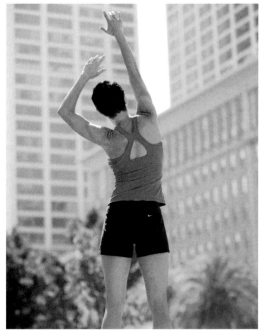

Torso stretch

CHAPTER 5

Phase 1: Building Your Base, Weeks 1 thru 4

Welcome to the first phase of your new fitness regimen! You've learned the fundamentals of Outdoor Fitness, including what it means to read—and interact with—your environment. You've taken the first steps in exploring the BodyMind connection and recognized the importance of mental clarity and emotional balance to your fitness regime and overall health. You've set personal goals, learned how to evaluate your terrain, and learned how to scout locations and select a safe, effective, interesting workout site. Now it's time to get outdoors and get to work at having some clean dirty fun!

I recommend that everyone—regardless of fitness level—begin with the workouts in Phase 1. In the three workouts that follow, you'll receive a hands-on introduction to the essentials of Outdoor Fitness:

• You'll work on body alignment and get used to setting up with strong posture—and keeping that posture as you exercise.

• You'll learn the powerful Base Moves that will be the core of all your workouts to come.

• You'll experiment with each of the basic types of workouts: single site, multisite, and traveling.

• You'll practice breathing techniques and integrate purposeful breathing into even your most strenuous routines.

• You'll implement BodyMind exercises and strategies throughout each workout to deepen your connection to nature and to your own "inner self."

• You'll preview the core of your core, a key component of Phase 2 and beyond.

All three workouts in Phase 1 can easily be adapted to suit all fitness levels, from the novice exerciser to the seasoned athlete. Throughout each session, you'll find suggestions for modifications to increase and decrease the difficulty of the exercises.

Workout 1 is a fun, manageable, single-site session that packs a lot of activity into a little time: It tones and strengthens your lower body and your core, and also builds joint strength, balance, proprioceptive awareness, and mental focus. Workout 2 gets you moving from station to station for your first multisite session, combining strength and toning with bursts of cardio. You'll love the fast pace and variety of this session—perfect for a grassy park or your high school athletic field. You'll start to really travel in workout 3, which builds full-body muscular strength and endurance and also offers great cardiovascular challenges.

By the end of your four weeks in Phase 1, you'll be well on your way to meeting your fitness goals. You'll have built muscle and core strength, and started to tone up your whole body. You'll have made great strides in your cardiovascular ability and made real improvements to your cardiovascular health. You'll be adept at reading your terrain, working with your environment, and tapping into your personal connection with the natural world. You'll be in touch with the quiet power of mindfulness and mental focus, and you'll be using this power to improve your whole health and well-being.

Are you excited? You should be, because you're about to start an empowering and meaningful journey, one that is going to transform your body and your mind.

Form and Alignment

Proper form and alignment are the foundation of every exercise. To be in good form means your body is in a strong, supportive position, from the soles of your feet to the crown of your head. This allows your frame (i.e., the skeletal segments of your body) to be properly aligned, with your muscles fully supporting your joints. By maintaining form and alignment, you create a strong core from which you can maximize your exercises and prevent injuries. Remember: Form and alignment are as important to each exercise as the movements themselves.

Form and alignment take on new dimensions when you're working out outdoors. The terrain outside is varied and ever changing. Rarely will you find terrain to be completely flat; there's usually a curve, undulation, incline, or decline. To keep your exercises effective and your body safe from injury, you need to stay aligned with the terrain underfoot.

Find the Fall Line

The natural downhill course of any slope is called the fall line. When you exercise outdoors, you're often working on ground that is not level. This is great for your body and your mind, but it requires that you make adjustments to align yourself properly, and safely, on uneven terrain.

When preparing for an exercise on outdoor ground, be sure to first analyze the fall line so that you can properly align your body on the uneven terrain. For example, when aligning for a squat on a slope, face the fall line—that is, face downhill—with your back to the uphill slope. Now distribute your weight evenly between both feet. To ensure that you don't slip, weight your heels more than your toes. If more pressure is applied through the forefoot, there's a very good chance you'll slide onto your behind!

Create a Base of Support

Outdoor terrain is full of variety—fall lines, textures, lumps, and bumps. To work effectively and safely on such var-iegated surfaces, you need to provide your body with a broader base of sup-port. Your base of support is your area of stability and includes the area of ground below the body that spans your body's points of contact.

To illustrate this, let's compare two types of squats: the traditional squat and the wide-legged squat. In the traditional squat your feet are positioned shoulder-width apart, with toes pointed forward. In a wide-legged squat your feet are placed well beyond shoulder-width, with your toes naturally angling out. Whether you're on a steep slope or just slightly uneven ground, you'll find the wider squat is more stable and comfortable due to its greater base of support.

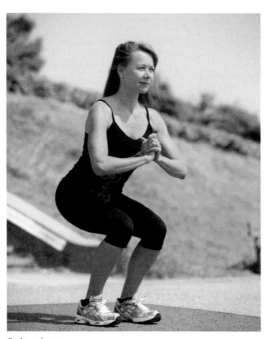

Traditional squat

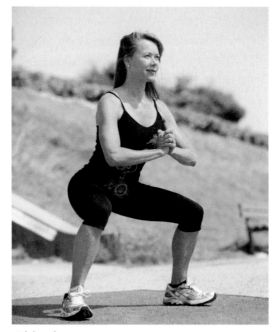

Wide-legged squat

Get into Proper Starting Position

There are two basic positions—or stances—that you will rely on throughout all your Outdoor Fitness sessions: the athletic stance and the split stance. Both positions provide you with a broad base of support for all your Outdoor Fitness moves, so you can work confidently and with full range of motion on any terrain.

Athletic Stance

- Stand with your feet shoulder-width apart, distributing your body weight evenly between both feet.

- Maintain a slight bend to your knees.
- Shoulders should be square, with your shoulder blades drawn slightly together to open your chest.
- Lightly lift your rib cage up to elongate your spine and to activate your abdominal wall for a little added support to your spine.

TIP: For added balance, keep your eyes focused forward, with your chin parallel to the ground.

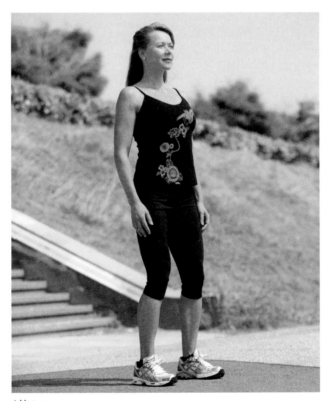

Athletic stance

Split Stance

The split stance not only offers a strong base of support, it also helps to prevent lower-back strain and enables you to work on the narrowest of trails with confidence.

- From the basic athletic stance, step back about 20 to 30 inches with one foot, and bend both legs to create a firm base of support.
- Keep your hips squared with your shoulders, with your hip bones pointing forward.
- Maintain the alignment of your upper body by keeping your shoulders square, your ribs lifted, and your abs taut.
- Distribute your weight evenly between the front heel and the rear toes.

> **TIP:** To avoid lower-back strain, keep your back straight and bend *slightly* at the hips to tilt your upper body forward.

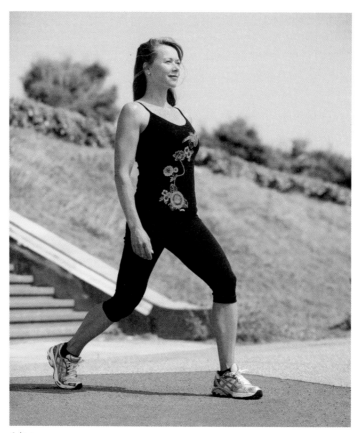

Split stance

Base Moves

Base Moves are the foundation of your Outdoor Fitness program, the "base" on which you'll build your strength, flexibility, endurance, and mental focus, from the inside out. These moves are designed to make you strong—physically, mentally, and emotionally—all while you're integrating with your outdoor environment. The strengthening and foundation they provide also help to keep you safe from injury.

Base Moves get your body moving the way it *wants* to move, the way it was *built* to move. Forward. Backward. Laterally. Diagonally. Squatting, lunging, bending, twisting, pushing, and pulling. Simple, elemental moves that you were born to do.

These 12 moves will get you in top form for a multitude of terrains and fun outdoor exercise sessions. When you work with Base Moves, you're not just training your muscles, you're also training your joints, balance, and mental focus. You'll get comfortable moving and flowing with the outdoor terrain. Before you know it, you'll be floating along the uneven terrain, moving up, down, forward, backward, and laterally, using your pushing, pulling, and lifting muscles. You'll feel your core—your deep stability muscles—getting stronger and leading the way.

Don't mistake Base Moves as beginner-only exercises. They're not. Nor will you want to leave them behind as you add new moves to your repertoire. These moves will challenge you, no matter what your starting fitness level and no matter how long you train. See Modifications—Harder, below each exercise, if you find that you'd like to "make it tougher" and increase the intensity and resistance.

Base Moves

- ☐ Wide-legged squat
- ☐ Split squat
- ☐ Standing forward lunge
- ☐ Reverse lunge
- ☐ Lateral leg press
- ☐ Calf raise
- ☐ Push-up
- ☐ "Reverse" pull-up
- ☐ Triceps dip
- ☐ Single-leg dip
- ☐ TVA/ab flattener
- ☐ Aqua

Wide-Legged Squat

This squat's wider stance is preferred for its greater control on uneven terrain and to target the inner thighs.

Works: Glutes, hamstrings, quadriceps, adductors, and balance.

Props: Flat ground.

Starting position: From the athletic stance, position your feet just beyond shoulder-width apart, with the toes positioned naturally from the heels. Distribute your body weight evenly between your feet. Lift your ribs and lower your shoulders, down away from your ears. Raising your hands to the height of your sternum, press your palms firmly together (what I call a "palm-to-palm press") to engage your center. Maintain this pressure between your palms.

Action: Inhale as you lower your hips, pressing your tailbone back behind you as your knees create a 45-degree angle. Be sure to keep your knees aligned over your feet and feel your body weight in your heels. Pause for a second, then exhale as you press up through your heels to the starting position.

MODIFICATIONS

Easier: Lower your hips only 2 to 3 inches.

Harder: Lower your hips until your knees create a 90-degree bend.

FOCAL POINTS

- For maximum effectiveness, emphasize drawing back the tailbone as if you are reaching for a chair behind you.
- Keep your spine aligned by lifting and engaging your midsection.

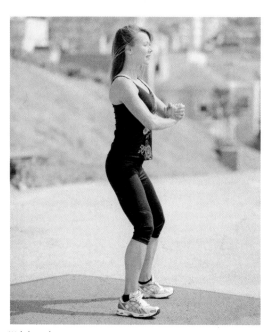

Wide-legged squat

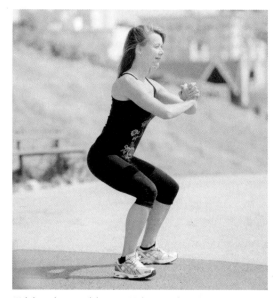

Wide-legged squat with knees at 45-degree angle

Split Squat

This is a time-efficient exercise that quickly strengthens and sculpts the legs and glutes. You are training the legs independently, where the front leg works the glutes and hamstrings while the back leg sculpts the quadriceps. Core strength and balance skills are also enhanced.

Start out practicing this exercise on flat ground, and then you can add a curb or step to place your back toes on for more challenge.

Works: Glutes, hamstrings, quadriceps, balance.

Props: A curb, root, berm, or step with a 3- to 8-inch rise.

Starting position: From the athletic stance, step back into a long split stance, resting your right foot—toes down, heel up. Place your hands on your hips and distribute your weight evenly between your front heel and the back toes.

Action: Inhale as you lower your hips until your left knee is at a 45-degree angle. Keep your eyes focused forward, your ribs lifted, and your shoulders square; don't collapse your upper body forward. Keep your bent left knee in line with your ankle and exhale as you press back up through your front heel and your back toes.

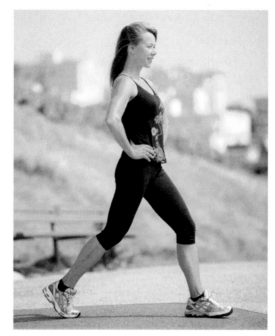

Split squat

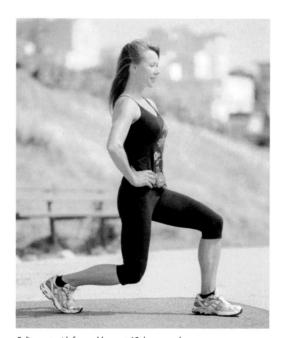

Split squat with forward knee at 45-degree angle

MODIFICATIONS

Easier:

- Perform this move on a flat surface.
- Steady yourself by holding on to a prop if you feel unstable.

Harder:

- Lower your hips until your forward knee is at a 90-degree angle.
- Place your back leg on a step, curb, or berm.

FOCAL POINTS

- If you find that your forward knee is wobbling, take control both mentally and physically.
- As you rise, contract your lower abdominal wall and press firmly into the ground through your forward heel.

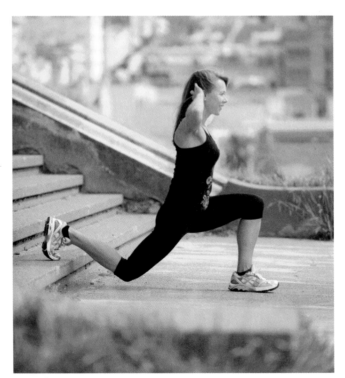

Split squat with prop

Standing Forward Lunge

Lunges are a staple of your Outdoor Fitness program because you can do them on a variety of terrain. Once you are comfortable with the basic forward lunge, you can progress by moving along grassy knolls and sandbars and up stairs, ramps, and hills. You can also incorporate fun props like stumps, curbs, and flat rocks for step lunges.

Works: Glutes, hamstrings, quadriceps, core stability.

Props: Flat ground.

Starting position: Start in the athletic stance, with your hands on your hips, ribs lifted, chest open, and eyes forward.

Action: Inhale as you take a long step forward onto your right foot so that your right knee forms a 45-degree angle and your left knee points down to the ground. Maintain even balance and weight distribution between both legs. Exhale as you engage your midsection, and push back through the right heel to the starting position. Repeat on the left leg.

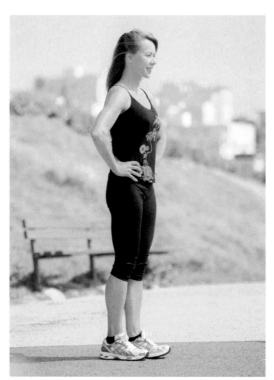

Athletic stance as starting position for standing forward lunge

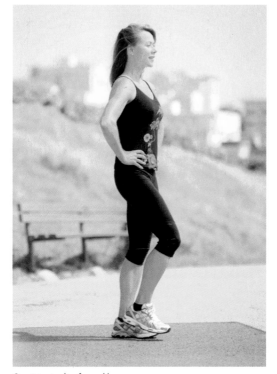

Step into standing forward lunge

MODIFICATIONS

Easier: Step forward with only a slight bend at the knee.

Harder:

- Bend your forward leg to a 90-degree angle.
- Work one leg for a full set, then repeat on the other leg for a full set.

FOCAL POINTS

- Keep your forward knee in line with your ankle.
- For added support and stability, engage your lower abdominal wall.

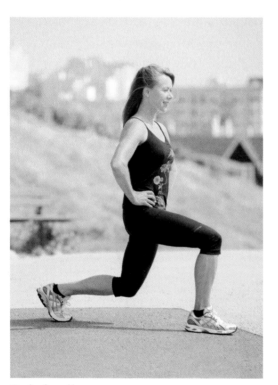

Standing forward lunge

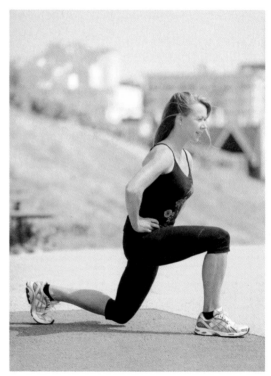

Standing forward lunge with forward knee at 90-degree angle

Reverse Lunge

The reverse lunge helps you gain strength, especially in your quadriceps. It will also rapidly improve your balance and spatial awareness in the ever-changing outdoor environment.

Works: Hamstrings, glutes, quadriceps, balance.

Props: Flat ground.

Starting position: Start in the athletic stance, with your hands on your hips, chest open, and eyes forward.

Action: Inhale as you take a long step backward onto your right toes so that your right knee points down to the ground. Gradually lower your hips until your left knee is bent at a 45-degree angle. Exhale as you press firmly through your back toes to the starting position. Alternate between the right and left legs.

MODIFICATIONS

Easier: Step back with only a slight bend in the forward knee.

Harder:
- Bend your forward knee to a 90-degree angle
- Do not alternate legs; work one leg for a full set, then switch.

FOCAL POINTS

Maintain even balance and weight distribution between both legs.

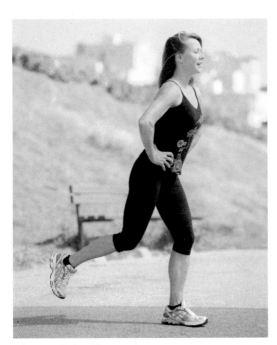

Taking a step backward for reverse lunge

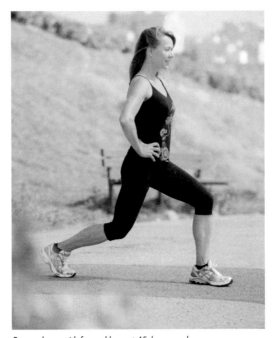

Reverse lunge with forward knee at 45-degree angle

Lateral Leg Press

This is an excellent exercise for the adductors of the inner thigh, as well as the abductors of the outer thigh and hips. Add an upper-body "palm-to-palm press" with your hands to improve posture and to engage and activate the core muscles. As you become stronger and more comfortable with the exercise, try it while traveling up ramps and hills, steps and stairs.

Works: Adductors, abductors, glutes, thighs.

Props: Flat ground.

Starting position: Begin with the athletic stance, and firmly press your palms together, keeping your elbows level.

Action: Take a wide step out laterally, onto your right foot; weight both feet evenly. Inhale, pressing your tailbone back, while lowering only slightly (no more than a 45-degree bend at the

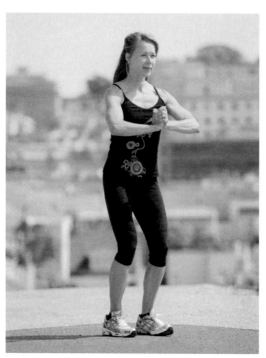

Starting position for lateral leg press

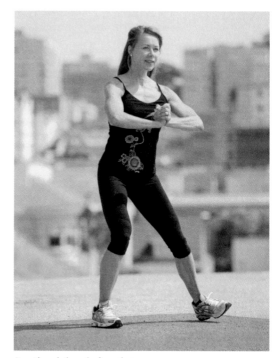

Press through the arch of your foot.

knees). Exhale as you press through the arch of your left foot—big toe to heel—back to the starting position. Continue moving laterally to the right for a series of two to eight steps, pressing firmly through the arch of the left foot—big toe to heel. Alternate between moving right and left.

MODIFICATIONS

Easier: Lower your tailbone no more than an inch or so.

Harder: Lower your tailbone to a 45-degree bend at the knees, and stay there! Do not stand up. Stay in this lower position throughout the entire exercise. (Remember, the lower your tailbone, the more challenging the move. So work your way "down" over time.)

FOCAL POINTS

- If there is even a slight incline, travel *up* the hill, not down it.
- Don't slip! No matter the terrain, make sure that you finesse and feel through your feet.
- Protect your lower back and engage your center for support by keeping your hands pressed firmly together at sternum height.

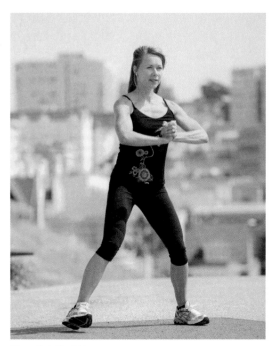

Step wide to the right

Calf Raise

Calves are a notoriously tough area to strengthen and tone. They are also an important muscle group that helps you balance and move more gracefully. Think about it: Calves do a lot to help us move and balance our bodies over the lumps and bumps in the terrain.

Works: Calves, balance, proprioception.

Props: Step, curb, tree root. (Safety tip: To avoid slipping, use only dry roots.)

Starting position: Starting from the athletic stance, place your toes and the balls of your feet along the edge of a curb, step, or tree root, hanging your heels over the edge.

Action: Inhale as you lower your heels and exhale as you lift your heels up, using a full range of motion in both directions.

MODIFICATIONS

Easier: Start with flat terrain until you feel balanced, or find something to hold on to for support.

Harder: Try these calf raises with your eyes open for half of the set, then try them with eyes closed.

FOCAL POINTS

• For added balance, find a focal point in the distance and stay focused on it.

• For greater stability throughout, engage your midsection and maintain good posture, with your hands in your peripheral vision.

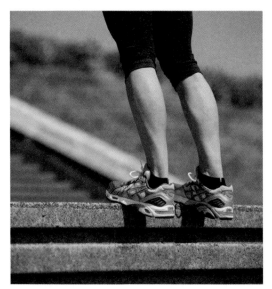

Calf raise, heels lowered

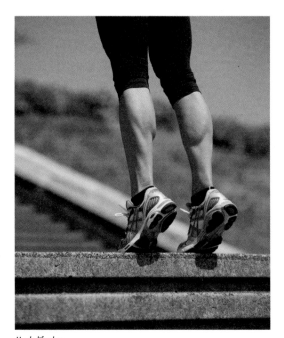

Heels lifted up

Push-Up

I think this is the best all-around upper body toner, because it not only works your chest muscles as primary movers, it calls upon your shoulders, arms, serratus muscles, and abdominals to play supporting roles.

Works: Pectorals, anterior deltoids, core stability.

Props: Bench, low wall, curb, log, boulder, or any flat surface.

Starting position: Place your hands on the prop just a bit wider than shoulder-width apart. Step back to a distance that elongates your backside in a straight line from your heels to your head.

Action: Inhale as you slowly lower your body until your midchest is a few inches from the prop. Pause. Exhale and press firmly through your hands back to the starting position.

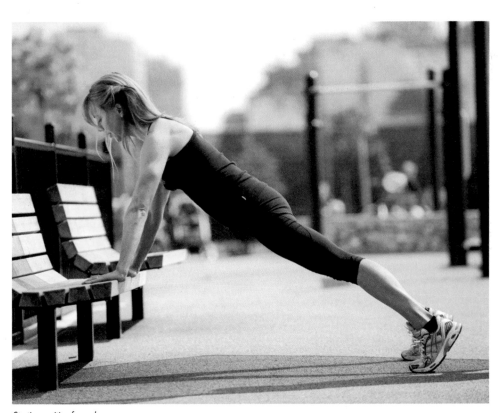

Starting position for push-up

MODIFICATIONS

Easier: Use a taller prop to lean on, like a wall, large tree, fence, or picnic table.

Harder: Use flat ground, or go inverted by placing your feet on a log, bench, or step, placing your hands on the ground.

FOCAL POINTS

- Don't sag in the spine; engage the abdominals for support.
- Keep your head in line with your spine.
- As you exhale up, imagine that your breath blows you back up to the start.

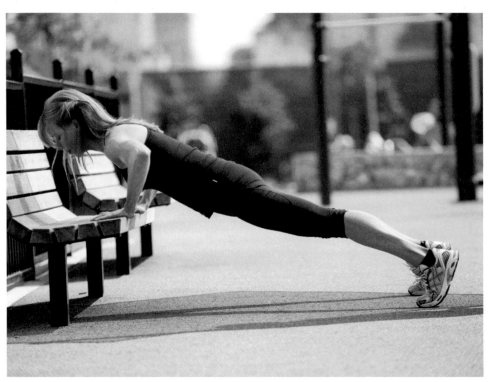

Chest lowered to prop

"Reverse" Pull-Up

A pull-up is tough, but reversing it so the lowering part is the resistance phase makes it easier and will strengthen your muscles just as effectively.

Works: Upper back, latissimus dorsi, deltoids, biceps.

Props: Low gate, monkey bar, or tree limb.

Starting position: Grip the bar or limb with your hands shoulder-width apart and your palms facing away from you. Walk your feet forward until your body is elongated and your knees are nearly straight, but not locked, balancing on your heels.

Action: Exhale as you pull yourself up until your chest touches, or nearly touches, the bar. Hold for one count. Inhale as you *slowly* lower your body back down until you feel the lengthening in your back muscles.

MODIFICATIONS

Easier:

• Get a little help from your legs by bending them and placing your feet a bit flatter.

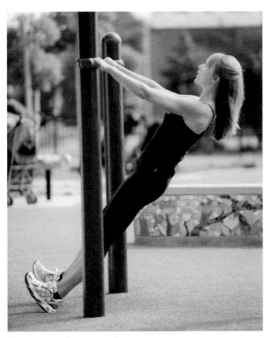

Starting position for reverse pull-up

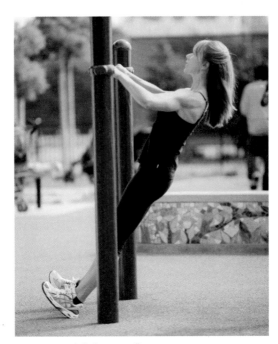

Maintain a straight body as you pull

- Remember, you'll get stronger by *slowly* lowering your body back to the start.

Harder:

- Select a prop that is just above the height of your head, such as a tree limb or a playground structure.
- Exhale as you pull your body up until your chin clears the limb.
- Inhale as you *slowly* lower back down.

FOCAL POINTS

- Work through full range of motion— pull all the way up to the bar or tree limb, and lower all the way down until you feel the stretch in your upper back.
- Emphasis is on a slower lowering phase of the movement.

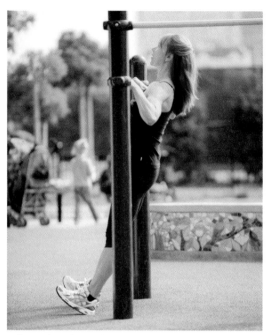

Pull up until your chest touches, or nearly touches, the bar

Triceps Dip

This exercise does an excellent job shaping your shoulders and your arms.

Works: Deltoids, triceps.

Props: Bench, log, stump, high step, concrete block.

Starting position: Take a seat on the edge of a bench or block. Place your palms, fingertips down, along the edge. Extend your legs in front of you, slightly bent, resting on your heels.

Action: Inhale and lower your hips until your upper arms are nearly parallel to the ground, then exhale back up, pressing firmly through your palms.

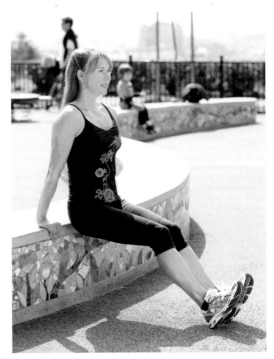

Set up for triceps dip

MODIFICATIONS

Easier: Use two flat feet and bend your knees.

Harder: Use only one heel for support and keep the other leg straight out from your body, with a hard flex to your foot (toes pointing toward the sky).

FOCAL POINTS

• Keep your shoulders square and down, away from your ears. Your tailbone should be just clearing the bench.

• Protect your rotator cuff—don't dip down below 90 degrees at the elbow.

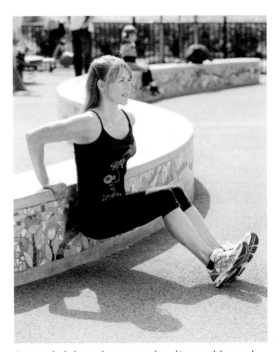

Keep your back close to the prop as you lower hips toward the ground

93

Single-Leg Dip

This is an excellent exercise for building proprioception and balance. It also does a great job at strengthening the ankle, knee, and hip joints.

Works: Hamstrings, quadriceps, glutes, joint stability, proprioception, balance.

Props: Flat ground.

Starting position: Stand firmly on the flat ground. Take a deep breath to get quiet and centered. Find a focal point in the distance and stay focused on that point. Next, ground down through your left foot and draw your right foot forward, about 12 to 15 inches off the ground. Bring your hands together into a "palm-to-palm press."

Action: Inhale as you bend your left knee, sinking down through your hips and balancing through your foot, aligning the center of your knee with your second toe. Exhale up, pressing through your big toe, little toe, and heel.

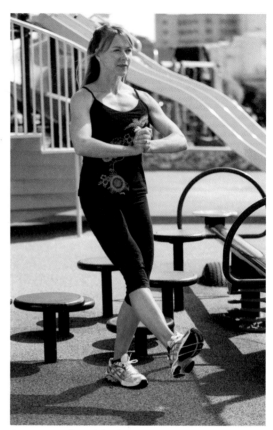

Starting position for single-leg dip

MODIFICATIONS

Easier:

• Bend your knee only an inch or 2.
• For added stability, hold on lightly to a prop, like a tree or bench.

Harder:

Lower yourself so that you bend your knee farther, but no more than 45 degrees.

FOCAL POINTS

• To avoid wobbling on the supporting leg, take control through the quadriceps.
• Align the center of your knee with your second toe.
• If you feel discomfort behind your kneecap, pressure your foot only from the midarch to the heel of your foot.

TVA/Ab Flattener

My clients swear by this exercise. They think TVA stands for Tina Vindum's Abs, when it really stands for the main muscle we are targeting: the transverse abdominus. The beauty of this abdominal muscle is that it lies deep within the core muscles. It's a "stability" muscle, which, if it's trained efficiently, can and will flatten that dreaded "pooch" that happens after pregnancy or through the natural effects of aging. Gravity and the process of living cause our innards to droop outward—thus, the pooch. But this is not your destiny. You can tighten the muscles just like a natural girdle, to pull everything back in, for a tight, flat abdominal wall—flat from the pelvis to the ribs!

Works: Transverse abdominus.

Props: Flat surface—picnic table, bench, grass, sand, concrete.

Starting position: Lie on your back with your hands held lightly behind your head, elbows pointing out to the side. Bend your knees and keep your feet flat and spaced shoulder-width apart, about 12 to 15 inches from your glutes. Press the area between your navel, your hips, and your tailbone firmly into the ground—and maintain this pressure throughout the entire exercise.

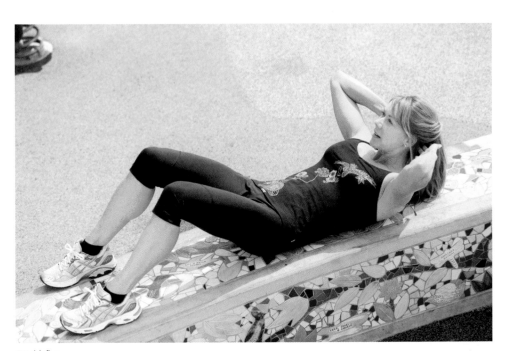

TVA/ab flattener

Action: Exhale, lifting your shoulder blades anywhere from ½ inch to 2 inches off the ground. Inhale as you lower. Maintain even pressure between your navel and the pelvis, and make sure your feet remain flat—toes to heel.

FOCAL POINTS

- Maintain even pressure from your navel through your hips, so that you're working the deep layers of your abdominal wall.
- Use your torso to do the work. Do not pull on your head to create momentum.

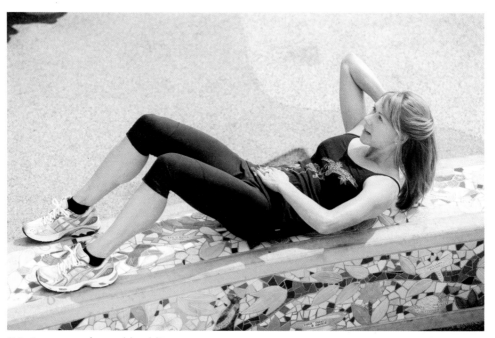

Maintain even pressure from navel through hips

Aqua

People think that abdominal work is enough to help prevent back injuries and improve posture. Not true. You also need to work the opposing muscle group, the erectors that line the spine.

Works: Back erectors, glutes, hamstrings, deltoids.

Props: Flat surface—picnic table, bench, grass, sand, concrete.

Starting position: Lie face down on the ground with your head in line with your spine. Lengthen your arms overhead, palms down on the ground.

Action: Lift your right arm and your left leg up, pause, then lower. Alternate, lifting your left arm and right leg. Continue, slowly lifting and lengthening your opposite arm and leg, as if you're swimming.

FOCAL POINTS

- Keep your head in line with your spine. Do not rest your forehead on the ground.
- With each lift, lengthen your arms and legs as if someone is pulling on them.

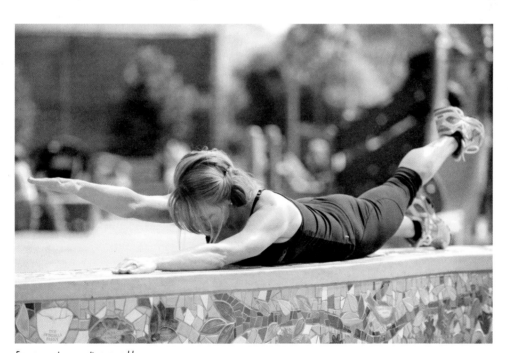

For aqua, raise opposite arm and leg

Workout 1: Single Site

> **WORKOUT SNAPSHOT**
>
> **Total time:** 30 minutes.
> **Props:** A 3- to 8-inch step, curb, low wall, or berm.
> **Location:** Just about anywhere.
> **Purpose:** Muscular strength and toning for your lower body and core. Multidirectional movement, joint strength, mental focus, proprioceptive awareness, and balance.

This workout is great for its versatility. You can take this session to the local park, a city plaza, a picnic area, the beach—or even your backyard. In scouting your terrain, you'll need a flat or semiflat spot with a berm, step, curb, or low wall nearby for step-ups and split squats. Note that near the end of the session, you'll need to lie back on the terrain. If your location doesn't give you that option, that's okay; just save the last two exercises for your floor at home. Before you get started, be sure to clear the area of any debris that you can slip on or trip over, such as branches, twigs, needles, gravel, or rocks.

Stage 1: Warm-Up (5 to 10 minutes)

Do your "one-spot warm-up" (see chapter 4), and then continue with the following (which are all described in chapter 4):

1. Joint lubrication
2. Reverse breath
3. Posture check
4. High knees
5. Step-ups

Stage 2: Multidirectional Strength Exercises (15 to 20 minutes)

It's time to start working with Base Moves, the rock-solid foundation of Outdoor Fitness. They will become your go-to exercises in the workouts to come, as well as the workouts you create yourself.

Detailed instructions on how to perform Base Moves can be found earlier in this chapter. Below you'll find coaching tips to get you started and keep you motivated, as well as modifications that will help you customize this workout to your current fitness level and your goals. Keep in mind that all the moves stem from your midsection or your center of mass. In the first four exercises, you will press your palms firmly together to enhance your posture and to engage your midsection.

Review of the Fall Line

The fall line is the natural downhill course of a terrain. It's important to adjust to the fall line so you can move safely and with full range of motion when working on a hill. To gauge the fall line, think about how a ball would roll or water would flow over the terrain. If you're aligning for a squat or other exercise, face down the fall line, with your back to the slope and your weight distributed evenly. Weight your heels more than your toes to keep from slipping.

The Wide-Legged Squat
(2 sets, 8 to 15 repetitions)

Preparation: Before performing your squats, scout the terrain for the most level section of ground. If there is even a slight slant, find the fall line and stand with your back against the uphill slope, your feet evenly weighted. Hands are in the palm-to-palm position for this exer-cise. Walk it out for 20 to 30 seconds between sets and before moving on to lunges.

MODIFICATIONS

Easier: Lower your hips only a couple of inches.

Harder: Lower your hips so your knee form a 90-degree angle.

Reverse Lunge
(2 sets, 8 to 15 repetitions)

Preparation: Scan the area—especially behind you—and remove any twigs, sticks, pinecones, slick leaves, and gravel. Start in the athletic stance with hands in a palm-to-palm position. Walk it out between sets and before moving on to lateral leg presses.

MODIFICATIONS

Easier: Step back with only a slight bend in the forward knee.

Harder:
- Step back so that your knee creates a 90-degree bend.
- Do not alternate legs. Work one leg for a full set, then switch.

Lateral Leg Press
(2 sets, 8 to 15 repetitions)

This exercise is all about the combination of power and finesse. Press firmly through the arches of your feet. At the same time, use your feet to feel all the textures of the terrain underneath you, so that you don't slip.

MODIFICATIONS

Easier: Don't lower your tailbone more than a couple of inches.
Harder: Lower your hips until you have a 45-degree bend at the knees. Stay in this lower position for the entire exercise.

Split Squat
(2 sets, 8 to 15 repetitions)

MODIFICATIONS
Easier:
• Perform this exercise on a flat surface.
• Hold on to a prop if you feel unstable.
Harder:
• Bend forward knee to create a 90-degree angle.
• Place your hands behind your head, elbows out to the side.

Calf Raise
(2 sets, 8 to 15 repetitions)

MODIFICATIONS

Easier: Start with flat terrain until you feel balanced, or find something to hold for support.
Harder: Do half of the set with your eyes open, and half with eyes closed.

The next two exercises develop core strength. You'll need a flat surface where you can lie down. Remember, you can do these at home if your site doesn't allow you to stretch out on the ground.

TVA/Ab Flattener
(2 sets, 10 to 25 repetitions)

Do one set, and then take a 20- to 30-second breather before performing the second set. When you are ready, flip over to perform the next exercise, which strengthens your backside and the muscles that line your spine.

Aqua (2 sets, 8 to 15 repetitions)
Stretch out your lower back by lifting your hips up and back and resting them on your heels. Reach your fingertips forward, alternating between your right arm and left arm, feeling the stretch in your shoulders and upper back.

Stage 3: Cooldown (5 minutes)

The cooldown phase of your workout is as important as the warm-up. By taking the time to cool down properly, you allow your body to unwind from its exertion, prevent stiffness and pain, and give yourself time to clear your mind before resuming your busy day.

Oxygen Energizer

- Slowly stand up. Check your posture. Take a series of three to six deep, energizing breaths.
- Stretch out your torso by reaching above your head with your right hand, then alternating with your left. Manipulate the stretch so that you feel it down the length of your torso.

Flexibility

Now move on to your cooldown stretches (see chapter 4):

- Hip flexors
- Hamstrings
- Quadriceps
- Adductors
- Calves

Workout 2: Multisite

WORKOUT SNAPSHOT

Total time: 30 to 45 minutes.
Props: Tree limb, low rung or bar, bench, log, low wall, or step.
Location: Local park, athletic field.
Purpose: Muscular strength and toning for your upper body; cardiovascular conditioning; proprioceptive awareness.

With multisite workouts, you're always changing things up! This session combines cardio, muscular strength, and toning in one quick, efficient session. This workout also incorporates mental focus and environmental integration techniques as you move between stations. You'll be busy with this one, challenged physically and mentally, and you'll cover more ground and add additional Base Moves to your repertoire.

This workout can easily be adapted to a number of locations: an open-air mall, the local athletic field, a stretch of beach, or a mountain trail. If you feel more comfortable doing so, go ahead and set up your strength stations in advance—otherwise, just play it by ear along the way. Just make sure the props are stable enough to handle your weight. You'll be stopping at each station for a couple of exercises and moving between stations at a moderate pace. For this workout you'll use a timer.

Stage 1: Warm-Up (5 to 10 minutes)

For descriptions of these exercises, see chapter 4.

1. Joint lubrication (1 minute)
2. Reverse breath (30–60 seconds)
3. High knees (1 minute)
4. Cardio warm-up (5 to 7 minutes)

> **TIP:** Use your warm-up as an opportunity to connect with your surroundings and activate your senses. What do you see? What do you hear? What do you smell? What are you aware of kinesthetically? Can you feel the pull of gravity? What textures can you feel around you, underneath you? Can you feel the contours of the earth through your feet?

Stage 2: Exercises

Perform two sets of each exercise, resting for 20 to 30 seconds between each set.

> **TIP:** Push-ups are a good core conditioner. The key is to activate and engage your midsection during both phases by slightly pulling in your abdominal wall.

Push-Up
(2 sets, 30 to 60 seconds)

Props: Bench, low wall, log, boulder, picnic table.

MODIFICATIONS

Easier: Use the incline of a wall or a large tree trunk.

Harder: Try these push-ups inverted, with your feet on the bench or low wall.

Cardio Walk or Jog
(2 to 3 minutes; RPE 7)

Take off and begin building your RPE up to an aerobic level of 7. Maintain your focus at least 10 to 15 feet in front of you, reading the terrain as it comes into view. Notice all the twists, turns, bumps, and cracks on the surface ahead of you

> **TIP:** Use this block of cardio to work on your environmental integration. Choose one or two types of sensory input (visual, aural, tactile, olfactory, etc.) and focus on these senses during your walk or jog.

and make contact with them by feeling through your feet. Focused and mindful of your environment, you can take the brakes off because you are prepared for what you will encounter.

As you approach time, bring your RPE down to a level 5, and keep an eye out for a gate, bar, or low branch for pull-ups.

RPE Review

RPE is the measurement of your perceived rate of muscular, cardiovascular, and psychological fatigue. It's an important tool for you to manage how hard you're working during your sessions. There are no wrong answers! Only you know how you're feeling. Your individual RPE helps you maximize efficiency during your workout. RPE runs on a scale from 1 to 10, weak to very strong.

At some point in your training, you'll find that walking doesn't do it for you anymore. You're making great progress! To get your RPE where you want it to be, you'll need to "shuffle." Something between a walk and a jog, shuffling feels like you are skimming over the terrain.

"Reverse" Pull-Up
(2 sets, 30 to 60 seconds or as many as you can do)
Props: Gate, bar, tree branch.

MODIFICATIONS
Easier: Bend your knees and allow your legs to assist you.
Harder: Use a higher bar or limb so your feet come off the ground as you lift and lower yourself.

Cardio Walk or Jog
(2 to 3 minutes; RPE 7)
Take your RPE to a 7 or 7.5 as you move toward your next station. Check in with your breathing, making sure that it is deep and complete, with an "easy in" and an "easy out." When you're about 30 seconds from time, take your RPE down to a level 5. Look for a spot to do your triceps dips.

Triceps Dip
(2 sets, 30 to 60 seconds)
Props: Bench, log, stump, or block.

MODIFICATIONS
Easier: Don't lower your hips very much, and keep your knees bent at about a 90-degree angle.
Harder: Place one heel on the ground and keep the other leg stick-straight, hip-height in front of you. Switch legs.

Environmental Integration and Sensory Awareness: The Core of Your Core

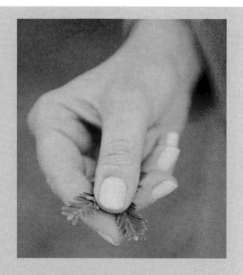

The practice of sensory awareness takes us to a place deep within ourselves. As you connect to everything that you see, hear, touch, smell, and even taste, you'll go deeper and deeper into what I call the "core of your core." You are so integrated with the environment that you become part of it, and it becomes part of you. It's a place where your senses become *so* heightened that it feels almost surreal. It's a mental and emotional high. It's a place of hyperconsciousness. It's very primal, and it's wonderful. When you get to the core of your core, you discover it's a place where you feel deeply alive, deeply grateful, and deeply connected to the world around you, and to your inner self.

Just like good balance and agility, enhanced sensory awareness is an acquired skill. To enhance your connection with your environment, stop at some point during your workout, close your eyes, and do the following:

- Feel the terrain underfoot. (This helps activate the nerves in your feet, bringing them on par with the nerves in your hands and helping you to step more surely as you walk.)
- Feel the pull of gravity.
- Take in the sounds around you.
- Feel the breeze brush your skin.
- Smell the aroma in the air.
- Listen to your internal voice.

Now as you continue to focus on these sense impressions, open your eyes and notice the colors and textures of your environment. Continue this exercise for several minutes before resuming your workout.

> **TIP:** Slower is better! Take your time going through your reps. Science has proven that you'll get more out of every bend and lift if you work slowly and mindfully through your exercises, because when you focus on the muscles you're working, you'll literally recruit more muscle fiber into the exercise.

Cardio Walk or Jog
(2 to 3 minutes; RPE 7)

Gradually take your RPE up to a level 7 or 7.5 and hold it there. Maintain your focus at least 10 to 15 feet ahead of you as you take in every color, texture, and sound. Imagine yourself becoming one with the environment as you feel the pull of gravity and the brush of the air against your skin. When you approach time, take your pace down and eventually walk it out for 30 seconds. You want your RPE at a 4 or less for your single-leg dips. Find a flat spot in the terrain to set up for your next exercise.

Single-Leg Dip
(2 sets, 30 to 60 seconds)

This is a proprioception/balance exercise, best done when you're breathing comfortably and feeling calm. If you feel fatigued, or if your heart rate feels high, walk for a bit until you feel relaxed and centered.

MODIFICATIONS
Easier:
- Bend your knee just an inch or 2 and make contact with both feet after each dip.
- For added stability, hold on lightly to a prop, such as a tree or bench.

Harder:
- Perform the exercise in slow motion: 3 counts down—pause—and 3 counts up.
- Start this exercise with your eyes open, then try it with your eyes closed.

Cardio Walk or Jog
(2 to 3 minutes; RPE 7)

On your return trip, build up your aerobic level to an RPE 7, working with oxygen. Breathe deeply and fully. Connect to the core of your core: You are calm, flowing along the trail, feeling at one with your surroundings, in harmony with your terrain. Enjoy this well-earned feeling!

TIP: Remember the mood-posture connection? It's impossible to feel low when you look up at the sky. Raise your head skyward and feel your mood lift!

Stage 3:
Cooldown
(5 to 10 minutes)

When you near your destination, gradually take your RPE down to a 3 or 4 by slowly jogging or walking for a couple of minutes. Keep an eye out for a quiet place to stretch and maintain this feeling of connectedness, peace, and well-being.

Flexibility

For descriptions of these stretches, see chapter 4.
- Hip flexors
- Hamstrings
- Quadriceps
- Chest
- Back
- Arms
- Shoulders

Workout 3:
The Traveling Workout

WORKOUT SNAPSHOT
Total time: 30 to 60 minutes.
Props: Tree limb, low bar or fence, log, bench, steps.
Location: A 1- to-5-mile course.
Purpose: Full-body muscular strength and endurance; cardio conditioning; mental focus.

This workout can last anywhere from 30 to 60 minutes since it's not guided by the clock but rather by your choice of destination. You choose the length of your route—and you can also choose its character! You might want to plot a solitary route on a day when you're feeling stressed, to make it easy to be alone with your thoughts, the rhythm of your breathing, and the sounds of nature. On the other hand, if you're feeling sociable, you might plot a route through the heart of town. Traveling workouts let you take a journey—and you can customize not only the physical terrain but also the mental landscape of your experience.

Along with muscular toning, this workout focuses on oxygen, or "energy training," to improve cardiovascular conditioning, muscular strength and endurance, mental focus, emotional power, and stress reduction. This is a cardio-based workout to a predetermined location where you'll do exercises that alternate between lower and upper body, giving your muscles a chance to rest in between. On the return trip you'll want to stay in your aerobic zone, working with oxygen, with an RPE of no higher than 7 to 7.5. (This is equivalent to 70 to 75 percent of your maximum heart rate.)

Stage 1:
Warm-Up and Cardio
(10 to 20 minutes)

This workout is heavy on cardio—but that doesn't mean you should shortchange your warm-up. You need to prime the circulation of oxygen through your body and brain, protect your muscles and joints from stress and strain, and initiate hormone release for carbohydrate and fat consumption.

For descriptions of these exercises, see chapter 4.

1. Reverse breath (30 to 60 seconds)

2. Joint lubrication (1 minute)

Start with your ankles, and move up your body to your shoulders. As you roll your shoulders back, lift your ribs, engage your center, and set your posture.

3. Fast walking (3 to 5 minutes)

Start walking, with a heel-toe roll and your high-toes technique. Feel the textures under your feet. Observe how your ankles are both strong and flexible. As you feel your heart rate slowly climb, use your arms to set your tempo.

4. Cardio fast walk or slow run to your location (10 to 15 minutes; RPE 7–7.5)

Take time to find a rhythm, settling in at RPE 7. Your breath should be steady but not gasping. At 7 RPE, you can talk, but you don't feel like it. Keep the muscles around your neck and shoulders loose and relaxed.

When you feel comfortable at this pace, bump it up to 7.5. This is your

It's All about Oxygen

Remember, you're working *with* oxygen in *your* aerobic zone—not my aerobic zone or your friend's aerobic zone! Be true to what you feel on the RPE 1–10 scale. You are oxygenating your system, burning fat, and toning muscles. If you move out of your aerobic zone, you will be working without oxygen, producing lactic acid in your muscles—and pushing too hard for this workout.

aerobic zone. As you increase your speed, relax your muscles and your mind. Pay attention to your environment. Take in the colors, textures, smells, and sounds. Read the path ahead of you and flow with the terrain—don't fight it.

When you arrive at your chosen location, walk it out for 30 to 60 seconds. If you are feeling tight, do some basic stretches. Outdoor exercisers tend to feel tightness in their hip flexors, hamstrings, and calves, especially when working on varied terrain. Go ahead and take a few moments to release any tension.

Stage 2:
Location Exercises
(10 to 15 minutes)

Repeat this sequence of exercises twice in the same order. Take a moment to feel proud of the work you're doing!

Shoulder and Hip Rotations
(30 to 60 seconds)

Loosen your upper and lower body. Take a moment to move your hips and shoulders through their full range of motion in both directions. Set your posture.

Wide-Legged Squat
(30 to 60 seconds)

Preparation: Set up on flat terrain.

MODIFICATIONS

Easier: Lower your hips only 2 inches.
Harder: Lower your hips so your knees form a 90-degree angle.

"Reverse" Pull-Up

Do as many of these as you can.
Props: Gate, bar, or tree limb.

MODIFICATIONS

Easier: Bend your knees and allow your legs to assist you.
Harder: Use a higher bar or limb so your feet come off the ground as you lift and lower.

Split Squat
(30 to 60 seconds per leg)

Props: A mound, low step, or root that is about 3 to 8 inches off flat ground.

> **TIP:** Focus on your lower body strength, core stability, and body balance. If you feel unsteady, stay with your focal point and imagine that you have a spotlight shining out from a spot just below your navel, and set your sights on the beam of light.

MODIFICATIONS

Easier: Perform this exercise on a flat surface. Hold on to a prop if you feel unstable.

Harder: Bend your forward knee to a 90-degree angle. Place your hands behind your head, elbows to the sides.

Push-Ups (30 to 60 seconds)

Preparation: Set up with a wide base of support, your feet at or just beyond shoulder-width apart. Make sure that you are level and centered on both the prop and the terrain. If you're cockeyed, you could tweak your shoulders.

Props: A bench, low wall, log, boulder, or curb.

MODIFICATIONS

Easier: Use a wall or large tree trunk.

Harder: Invert, with your feet on the bench or low wall.

Lateral Leg Press (1 to 2 minutes)

Preparation: Do these presses either on a flat surface or up an incline.

MODIFICATIONS

Easier: Don't lower your tailbone more than a couple of inches.

Harder: Lower your hips until your knees make a 45-degree bend. Stay in this lower position throughout the entire exercise.

Triceps Dip
(30 to 60 seconds)

As you become stronger, lengthen your legs more and more, always maintaining a slight bend to your knees. As your arms get fatigued, your body wants to put the weight into your legs. Do your best to keep your tailbone close to the bench during the entire exercise.

MODIFICATIONS

Easier: Lower your hips just slightly. Keep your knees bent at about 90 degrees.

Harder: Place one heel on the ground and keep the other leg stick-straight, hip-height in front of you. Switch legs.

Single-Leg Dip
(30 to 60 seconds per leg)

Cardio Return Trip:
Walk or Jog with a Moving
Meditation (10 to 15 minutes)

Props: Find a flat spot to stand. Take a few deep breaths to calm your body and mind.

As you run or walk back, take this opportunity to tune in to your mental focus by identifying your trigger thoughts: the places your mind is conditioned to go, the scenes and scenarios you play out in your thoughts. Replace them with a mindful focus on the present task.

Thoughts Are Things

You get what you think about. Your thoughts have the power to calm you down or stress you out. This has immediate physical consequences for your body. An anxiety-producing thought can increase your heart rate by five beats per minute. Conversely, calming thoughts can slow your heart rate by five beats.

Think about biting into an icy cold cluster of plump pomegranate seeds or sinking your teeth into a tart cherry. Did you feel the sensation of your mouth watering? That's how powerfully connected our thoughts are to our bodies. If a simple thought can do that, think of the effect that negative "what if" thoughts can have. During a walk, jog, or other rhythmic exercise, get into the flow of "low and slow" breathing. When you exhale, repeat these powerful and positive words: "I am fit, healthy, and vibrant."

Stage 3: Cooldown (5 minutes; RPE 6)

Walk it out to lower your RPE to 6 and wind down from your workout. You may want to wrap up your session with a positive mantra like, "I am fit, healthy, and vibrant!" Take a few deep, purposeful breaths and repeat your mantra as you exhale.

Flexibility (3 to 5 minutes)

For descriptions of these stretches, see chapter 4.
• Hip flexors
• Hamstrings
• Quadriceps
• Calves
• Inner thighs (adductors)
• Chest, shoulders, and biceps
• Back
• Upper back and rear shoulders

CHAPTER 6

Phase 2: Core of Your Core, Weeks 5 thru 8

Are you ready for some new challenges? Phase 2 is full of them! You're going to build on all the great work you've accomplished in Phase 1 to take your fitness regimen—and your overall health and well-being—to new heights. In the next four weeks, you will build on the physical skills and strength you've developed since you started Outdoor Fitness. You'll get stronger and faster. You'll increase your coordination, balance and agility, and kinesthetic and proprioceptive awareness. You'll continue to develop your mental acuity, becoming more adept at controlling your moods and pinpointing your focus. You'll try out new terrains, deepen your sensory awareness, and challenge yourself with more rigorous—and results-driven—moves.

In this phase you'll learn a whole new set of strength exercises. These Signature Moves build directly on the Base Moves you're already using, adding pieces to them to create "compound exercises" and "combination moves," which team your upper and lower body to recruit more muscle and burn more calories. They get your body moving across many planes of motion: up, down, forward, backward, laterally, and diagonally, twisting and rotating. You'd never get this kind of full-body engagement on the machines in your old gym. They're great for your mind, too, since they require moment-to-moment focus. Because these exercises are so efficient, you actually can spend less time working out!

Workout 4 is a fun, exciting single-site session, full of ups and downs, and it's one of my absolute favorites. You'll take this workout to a set of steps or stairs, where you'll challenge your cardio strength and your muscular strength and endurance—you'll also really work on balance and agility, as well as your core. Workout 5 goes into the heart of your city or town for a chance to try an urban session that will change the way you look at your opportunities for fitness in the city. In this multisite workout, great cardio segments in between stations build both upper and lower body muscular strength and endurance. Workout 6 gets you back on the road again for a traveling workout that works great in a rural area, but it also can be done along a path or a loop in your local park. Core and full-body strength combine with cardio and muscular strength and endurance in a classic traveling workout that you'll use again and again.

Signature Moves

Signature Moves add a whole new dimension and challenge to your Outdoor Fitness routine. These strength exercises are incredibly effective—and efficient—because they demand that your body work across multiple planes of motion. They are also great for mental focus: The challenge of multidirectional movements means you must be mindful every moment.

Signature Moves target your upper and lower body together, which increases the activation of more muscle fiber and stability from your center of mass and core. You'll find that doing your abdominal work outdoors not only feels better, it looks better, too! When was the last time you gazed up into a grove of trees or a blue sky with white puffy clouds, or when did you last feel the sunshine on your face as you performed your crunches? This is a vantage point that changes everything—not only your abs, but also your attitude about them. Core conditioning is essential not only for getting those flat abs you want, but also for maintaining a strong body and protecting your spine.

These moves also increase your heart rate, giving you new cardiovascular challenges. After you've created a strong fitness foundation with Base Moves, Signature Moves will take your workouts—and your overall health—to new levels.

You can't get this kind of fitness boost in a gym. These 22 creative and effective exercises are designed to be performed outdoors (without mirrors, thumping music, or distractions like TV and machines), using the natural and man-made "props" you encounter during your workout. These exercises turn the world into your portable gym: Each exercise requires no equipment and can be done anywhere, anytime, no matter how busy your schedule.

These exercises are also appropriate for your Phase 2 fitness level. As with Base Moves, you'll find modifications to the Signature Moves, and you'll also find tips for making the most out of each move.

Signature Moves

- ☐ Hill squat
- ☐ "Half-tuck" squat
- ☐ Sumo squat
- ☐ Diagonal stride
- ☐ Full-body lunge
- ☐ Parking meter press
- ☐ Tree sit
- ☐ Tree stand—lower body
- ☐ Tree stand—upper body
- ☐ One-armed press
- ☐ "Palm-to-palm" pull-up
- ☐ "Push it–pull it"
- ☐ Full-body press
- ☐ Full-body triceps dip
- ☐ Rock-n-balance
- ☐ Root raise
- ☐ TVA/march
- ☐ Monkey-bar curl
- ☐ Standing "C" crunch
- ☐ Standing cross-over crunch
- ☐ Standing oblique crunch
- ☐ Aqua pulse

Hill Squat

These are my favorite squats on the planet! Believe it or not, a hillside provides a stable and effective platform for working the glutes and hamstrings, especially the area where the two meet—that's the "high and tight" effect. You'll never get this kind of result doing squats on a gym floor.

The wider stance when coupled with the angle of the hill shifts your line of gravity farther back, allowing you to press farther back through the tailbone, stretching the inner thighs (adductors) and putting them through the eccentric (or stretch) phase, which is effective for toning that hard-to-reach area.

Works: Glutes, hamstrings, adductors, balance, environmental integration.

Props: A sloping section of grass, sand, dirt, sidewalk, or ramp.

Starting position: From the basic athletic stance, position your feet slightly beyond shoulder-width apart, with your toes angling outward from your heels. Align your body with the fall line—facing down the slope, with your body weight distributed evenly between both heels.

Action: Inhale as you lower your hips, pressing your tailbone back as far as you can (without collapsing at the waist) and keeping your knees aligned over your ankles. Lower your hips so your knees form a 45-degree angle.

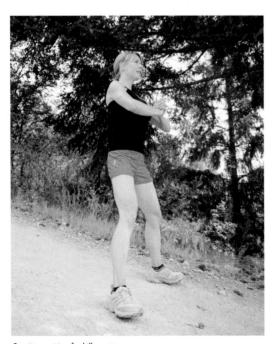

Starting position for hill squat

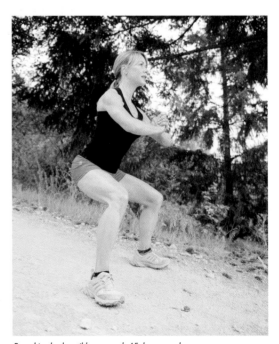

Press hips back until knees reach 45-degree angle

Pause for a moment. Exhale as you press up through the heels to the starting position.

MODIFICATION

Harder: Lower until your knees are at a 90-degree angle.

FOCAL POINTS

• The wider stance gives you greater control on uneven terrain and helps target the inner thighs.

• Use the forces of gravity to your advantage—slowly lower your hips to the count of 3, and slowly return to the count of 3.

• The more firmly you press through your heels, the more you'll work your glutes and hamstrings.

• When you add an overhead reach to this exercise, you'll activate your upper body and core—increasing caloric burn.

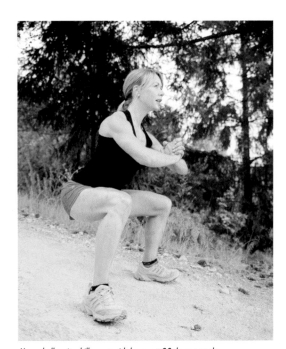

More challenging hill squat with knees at 90-degree angle

"Half-Tuck" Squat

Want to target that hard-to-reach inner-thigh area? Looking for a great move to strengthen your knee joint? I developed this exercise for just that purpose—and found that it also really toned my inner and outer thighs.

I call this a "half tuck" because you are isolating one leg at a time in a tuck position. The perfect location for this exercise is beside a short hillside or slope that typically lines the sides of a single-track trail, a fire road, or a paved path through a park. It also works great along a curb or parking block.

Works: Adductors, glutes, quadriceps, hamstrings.

Props: Hillside, curb, step.

Starting position: Using the side of a hill or grassy incline, prop your right foot laterally (sideways) on the slope of the hill so your foot is resting on the heel. Your leg should be straight but not locked. You may need to hop an inch or 2 to the left to line up your left foot on the flat surface of the trail or path.

Action: With your palms held together in front of you for counterbalance, press your tailbone back and lower until your left knee forms a 45-degree angle with the majority of your body weight on

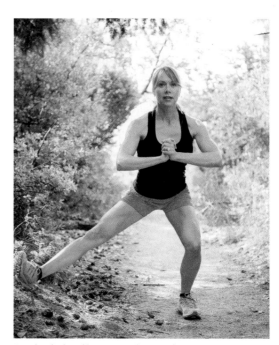

Starting position for half-tuck squat

Press hips back until knee is at 45-degree angle

your left leg. Inhale and sink downward, placing pressure on the entire bottom of your left foot, from the big toe to the heel. Exhale as you press firmly through the arch of your left foot to activate the adductors (inner thigh muscles) and push yourself back to the starting position.

MODIFICATIONS

Harder:

- Lower your hips until the bend of your knee is greater than a 45-degree angle.
- Get your chest out over your thigh and hold the tuck for 2 to 3 counts before returning to the starting position.

- Add a slight "tailbone-bob" (lifting and lowering your tailbone ½ to 1 inch) at the bottom of the move before you press back up to the starting position.

FOCAL POINTS

- Your resting leg should remain nearly straight, but not locked. It has no function in this exercise. You are just getting it out of the way.
- Do not let your knee drop beyond your toes. Keep your hips back.

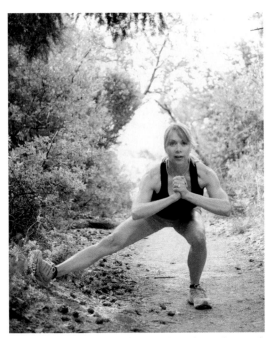

For harder half-tuck squat, lower until knee is deeper than 45-degree angle

TIP: This exercise is challenging, yes. That's because it requires total commitment and focus from you. When it's done correctly, you are loading your thigh with basically all of your body weight. Make sure that you maintain a solid knee throughout. Do not let it wobble. You can control a wobbly knee by tightening your abdominal wall on the way down and by mentally focusing on keeping your knee still.

Sumo Squat

Think Japanese sumo wrestler! The sumo squat is a wider variation of the wide-legged squat—ideal for when you're moving laterally over the terrain. I really like these squats because they're extremely effective for sculpting the inner and outer thighs as well as the hips and glutes. My clients love them because they're fun to do.

This exercise couples your upper and lower body, activating the deep muscles of the core. You can do sumo squats anywhere—in one spot on flat ground or across a hillside. To reap even greater cardio benefits, travel up a ramp, hill, or stairs.

Works: Glutes, abductors, adductors, quadriceps, hamstrings, deltoids, core, cardio.

Props: Flat ground, hills, steps, or stairs.

Starting position: From the athletic stance, take a wide step out laterally, onto your right foot, distributing your weight evenly between both feet.

Action: Inhale as you lower your hips, pressing your tailbone back, while at the same time lifting your arms diagonally, out and away from your body, palms in a fist, facing up. Lower into a wide squat until your knees create a 45-degree bend and you feel a lengthening of the inner thigh. Exhale as you return to the starting position by press-

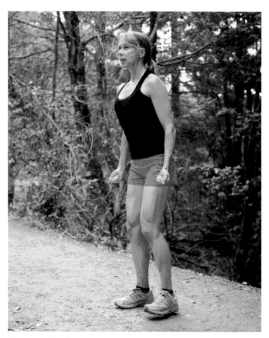

Starting position for sumo squat

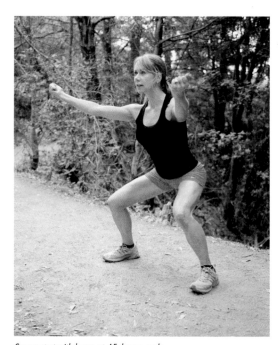

Sumo squat with knees at 45-degree angle

ing up through the left arch and lowering your arms. Repeat on the left leg, then alternate between the right and left legs.

Variation: Full-body traveling sumo squat. Follow the directions for sumo squats, only continue to move right for a series of 8 to 20 squats, pressing firmly through the arch of your left foot. Then travel back for a series, leading with the left.

MODIFICATION

Harder:

Lower until you create a 90-degree angle at the knees.

FOCAL POINTS

- Emphasis is on pressing your tailbone back, and then pushing up through the arch of the working foot to the starting position.
- Lifting your arms is more than a shoulder exercise when you concentrate on impeccable form—lifting your ribs to activate your center of mass, keeping your shoulders in line with your hips. Creating a fist will automatically pull in more muscle fiber in your upper body and remind your physiology to stay strong and in control.
- If there is an incline, always travel up the slope of the hill.

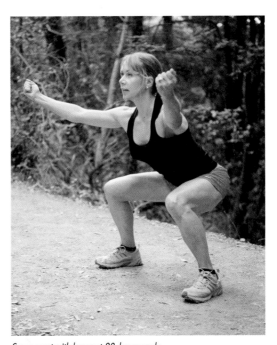

Sumo squat with knees at 90-degree angle

Diagonal Stride

Think skater and get low to use your glutes and legs for this powerful exercise. Don't let momentum do the work here.

Works: Glutes, abductors, adductors, calves, balance.

Props: Inclines, ramps, hills, stairs.

Starting position: Facing up the hill, take a long step up the hill with your right foot, into a diagonal stride—with your left elbow forward and in line with your right knee.

Action: Lean into the hill, with your body weight evenly distributed between both feet. Slowly lower your hips until you can feel pressure under the heel and arch of your right foot and the big toe and ball of your left foot. Exhale as you press off the big toe and the ball of

your left foot to engage the adductors of the inner thigh. Step your feet together, and alternate with the other leg, using your arms to set the tempo and to assist you with power in your stride.

MODIFICATION

Harder: As you lift, move more quickly, brushing the lifted knee and ankle just past the support leg.

FOCAL POINTS

• Face uphill.
• Lead with your forward foot.
• Move across the fall line in a zigzag fashion.

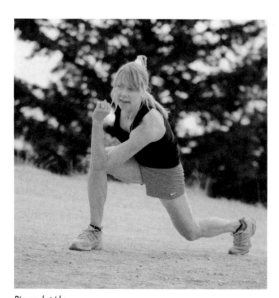

Diagonal stride

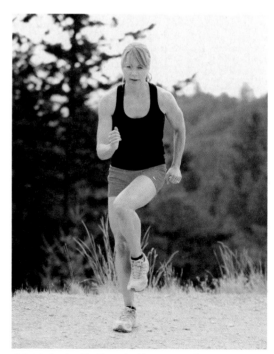

Mid-stride, brushing lifted leg and ankle past support leg

Full-Body Lunge

I created this exercise to give you the most value for your time. I believe it is the single most effective body-toning exercise you can do. By adding a few simple arm and leg movements to a walking lunge, you're working virtually every muscle from head to toe—as well as training your balance, coordination, and mental focus. Want even more? Try it on a slight incline or in soft sand—wow!

Works: Glutes, hamstrings, adductors, quadriceps, calves, hip flexors, abdominals and core stability, deltoids, triceps, balance, kinesthetic awareness, mental focus.

Props: Flat ground or slight incline.

Starting position: Stand tall, with your arms out to the sides at shoulder height and your hands balled into fists.

Action: Tighten your abs as you take a long step forward onto your left foot, so that your left knee forms a 45-to-90-degree angle and your right knee is pointed down toward the ground. At the same time, draw your fists (as in a pendulum swing) to your shoulders. Inhale as you sink down, maintaining even balance and weight distribution between both feet. Next, exhale as you push through your right toes, drawing your right knee up and away from your body and up toward your chest (forming the letter C with your abdominal

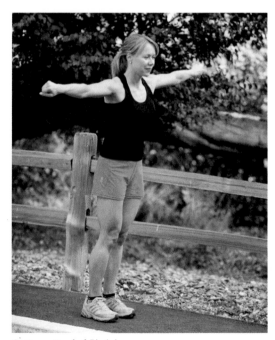

Starting position for full-body lunge

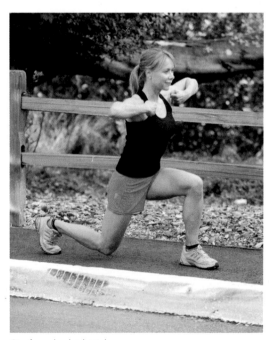

Step forward and sink into lunge

wall). At the same time, press your fists out to your sides, keeping them at shoulder height. Pivot up onto your left toes, with your arms straight out. Hold for one count before repeating with the opposite leg. Continue traveling as you alternate legs.

MODIFICATION

Harder: Bend your forward knee to 90 degrees.

FOCAL POINTS

- Maintain your elbows at shoulder height.
- Take control of your knees, mentally and physically, so they don't wobble.
- To maintain your form when pivoting up onto your toes, concentrate on contracting your glutes.
- Protect your lumbar spine during lunge portions of the exercise by tilting forward slightly at the hips.

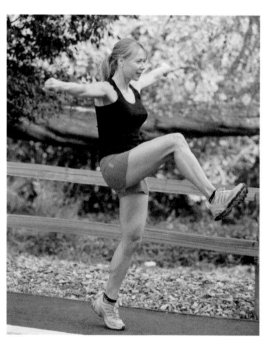

Rise up for another step

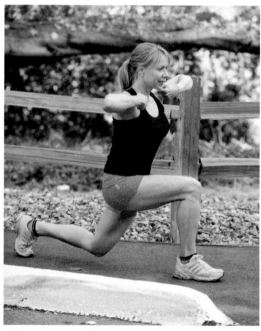

Sink into lunge on opposite knee

Parking Meter Press

Live in the heart of the city? Want to give your rear view a lift? I created this exercise for just this purpose. As you do it, think "high and tight"—and I'm not talking haircuts!

I call this exercise the parking meter press, but in reality it can be done virtually anywhere, with a variety of props. In the mountains I use trees. At the beach I use the lifeguard stand. You can also use playground structures, stop signs, flag poles, and fence posts.

Works: Glutes and hamstrings—intensely!

Props: Parking meter, post, tree.

Starting position: Wedge the ball of your left foot up against the base of the meter by bracing your toes against the pole so that your heel is planted firmly on the ground. Standing straight, lace the fingers of both hands around the pole at the height of your navel. Hook your right foot around your left ankle and keep it off the ground.

Action: Sit back as far as you can, so that your arms are straight and your

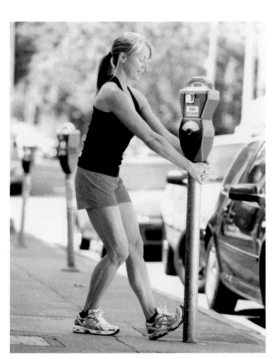

Starting position for parking meter press

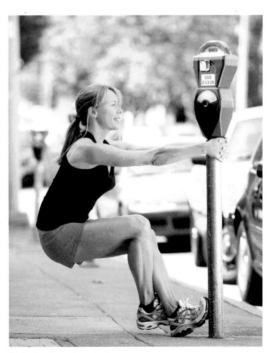

Sit back with weight on heel

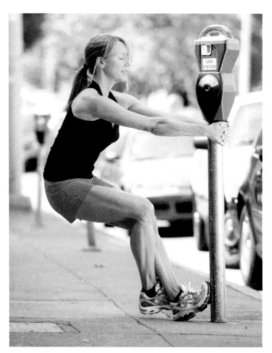

Press up through heel

left knee forms about a 45-degree angle. With your left heel supporting all your weight, press up through it, allowing your tailbone to rise only about 3 to 4 inches before you slowly return to the starting position.

MODIFICATIONS

Harder:

• Bend your knee to 90 degrees.

• Extend the time and the repetitions.

• Slow your tempo down: 3 counts down and hold, 2 counts up.

FOCAL POINTS

• The movement is small and precise—be sure not to collapse at the knee.

• Remember not to assist with your arms, as arms have nothing to do with this exercise.

TIP: Be sure to support yourself through your heel and not with your arms. By pressing firmly through your heel and leaning away from the pole, you ensure that you're working the correct area—the spot where your glutes and hamstrings come together.

Tree Sit

The tree sit exercise is an updated version of that classic ski-conditioning exercise, the wall sit. It's usually done within the confines of large gymnasiums with wood floors and beige walls, but here I've added a much more interesting prop—the tree. In addition to the tree's tactile nature, I also like the metaphor of gaining strength and power from the tree. Plus, while the classic wall sit only strengthens the quads, my version strengthens and tones the quads (in a big way), and it also works the deep muscles of the core and abdominals, and the shoulders. That's because you mentally focus on first pressing down through your heels, which gives you the leverage to press into the tree and engage your core.

Works: Quadriceps, core abdominals, shoulders, mental focus, environmental integration.

Props: Tree with a strong base, light post, wall, or mailbox.

Starting position: Find a strong tree with a circumference of at least 20 inches and a flat area around its base. You may also use a wall or a thick post—anything solid that you can lean against. To prevent your feet from slip-

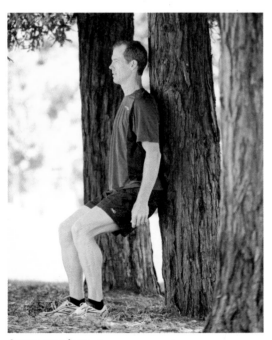

Starting position for tree sit

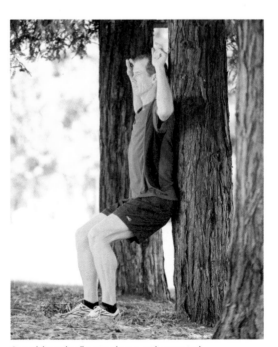

Press abdominal wall against the tree, with arms raised

ping, clear away any twigs, gravel, or debris first.

Action: Have a seat with your back up against the tree and your knees bent at a 45-degree angle. With your arms by your sides, press your heels firmly into the ground. Using the power from your heels and leverage from the tree, press your lower abdominal wall firmly into your lower back and up your entire spine. Hold your arms out to the sides at shoulder height, palms forward, and then bend your elbows so arms are at a 90-degree angle. Notice how your

entire abdominal wall is engaged and your chest opens.

MODIFICATION

Harder: Bend your knees at a 90-degree angle and march your feet in place.

FOCAL POINTS

- Keep your weight in your heels.
- Utilize your core for stability.
- Keep your hands off your thighs.
- To stand up, push off the tree with your hands to avoid straining the lower back.

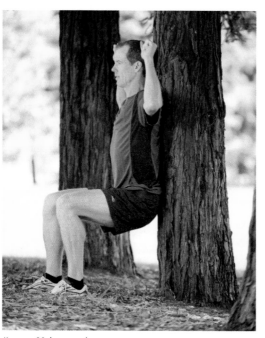

Knees at 90-degree angle

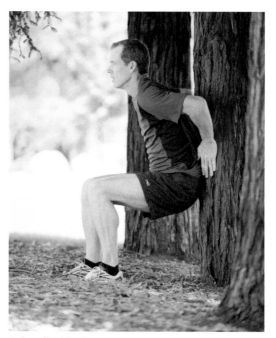

Pushing off with hands

Tree Stand— Lower Body

I like to encourage my clients to "touch" and be touched by nature in as many ways as possible (remember that "road rage" study using the calming scent of grass?).

This exercise concentrates on a number of things at once—posture, core stability, leg and gluteal toning, and mental focus. As you set up for the exercise, make sure that you are focused on good posture—head in line with your spine, hips squared with your shoulders.

Works: Core, glutes, hamstrings, balance, proprioception.

Props: Tree, post, wall, boulder.

Starting position: This exercise has you facing a tree, fence, or post that's about 3 to 4 feet away. Keeping your hips squared with your shoulders, bend over until your back is parallel to the ground. Extend your arms to *lightly* hold on to the tree and lift your right leg off the ground.

Action: Lengthen your body out so that you create the letter T; keep your legs, arms, and torso straight. Lift your right leg up and down a few inches to work the glutes.

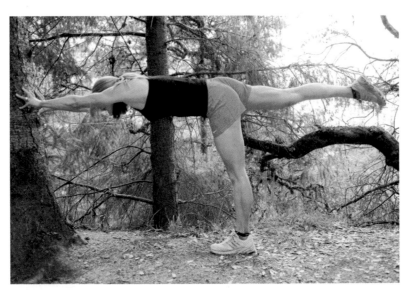

Starting position for tree stand—lower body

MODIFICATION

Harder: Bend your right knee at a 90-degree angle and press your heel to the sky, lifting and lowering.

FOCAL POINTS

- Tighten glutes for stability.
- Rely on your core, not the tree.
- Press lightly through the fingertips.

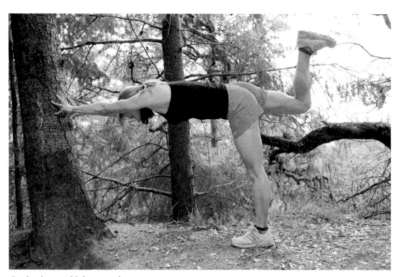

Bending knee at 90-degree angle

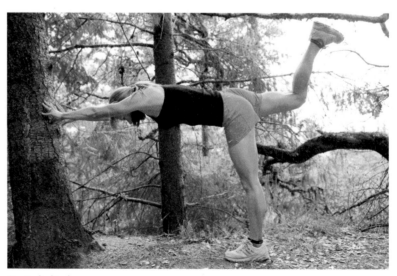

Pressing heel to sky

Tree Stand—Upper Body

You'll have fun with both the uniqueness and the effectiveness of this exercise because it won't take long to get the hang of it, and you can immediately feel how it trains your balance and tones your entire backside!

Works: Core, back, shoulders, glutes, hamstrings, balance, proprioception.

Props: Tree, post, wall, boulder.

Starting position: Stand with your back to a tree that's a few feet away. Keeping your hips squared with your shoulders, extend your arms overhead and lift your left leg off the ground, reaching it back for the tree's surface.

Action: Lengthen your body out, so that you create the letter T. Keep your left leg, arms, and torso straight. Lower your arms so your hands are facing in, balled into fists. Exhale as you raise your arms out to the sides, performing a reverse fly—isometrically squeezing your shoulder blades together.

MODIFICATION

Easier: Use a bent leg propped up against the tree.

FOCAL POINTS

- Maintain a light touch through your toes against the tree.
- Rely on your core, not the tree.
- Use mental focus to recruit maximum muscle fiber in your upper back.

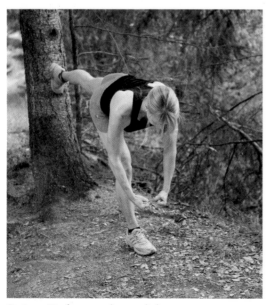

Starting position for tree stand—upper body

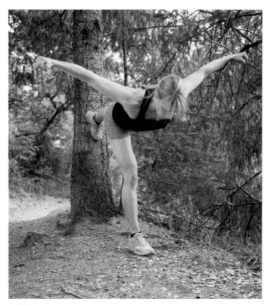

Raising arms

One-Armed Press

This exercise is a powerful arm, chest, and shoulder strengthener. It isolates one side of your body at a time for independent arm strength, which also helps to correct muscular imbalances.

Works: Pectorals, deltoids, triceps.

Props: Tree, fence, wall, back of bench, or table.

Starting position: From a standing position, place one hand sideways (elbows out) on the tree or fence at heart height and lean into it with all your body weight, allowing your heels to come off the ground. Step back to a distance that elongates your backside in a straight line from your heels to your head.

Action: Inhale and slowly lower until your chest is 3 to 5 inches away from your hand. Exhale as you press through your palm to the starting position. Repeat with the other arm.

FOCAL POINTS

- Avoid a sagging spine by engaging the abdominals for support.
- For extra power, imagine that your breath blows you back up into position as you exhale.

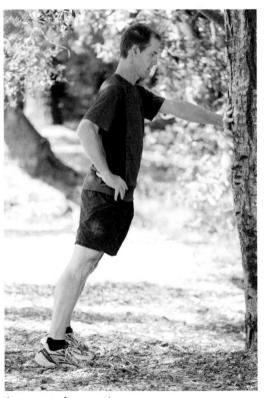

Starting position for one-armed press

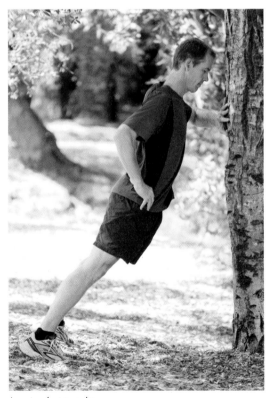

Lowering chest toward tree

"Palm-to-Palm" Pull-Up

This is a much easier version of the classic pull-up.

Works: Latissimus dorsi, the large "pulling" muscles of your back—trapezius, teres, rhomboids, deltoids, biceps.

Props: Tree limb or monkey bar.

Starting position: Select a prop that is just above the height of your head, such as a tree limb or a playground structure. Hang with your fingers laced together around the prop.

Action: Exhale as you pull yourself upward to your right shoulder and until your chin rises above the limb. Inhale as you slowly return to the starting position. Repeat, alternating between the right and left shoulder.

MODIFICATION

Easier: Place one foot against the tree or bar, or on a rock, for assistance.

FOCAL POINTS

• Exhale as you lift for power.
• Use full range of motion.

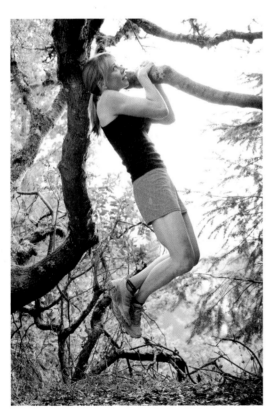

Palm-to-palm pull-up

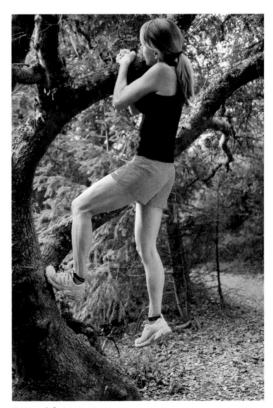

Easier with foot against tree

"Push It–Pull It"

Push-ups are an excellent, all-around toner and strengthener. This "push it–pull it" builds on the push-up by adding a one-armed row that pulls in your back muscles.

Works: Pectorals, deltoids, latissimus dorsi, rhomboids, triceps, core.

Props: Flat ground, step, bench, tabletop.

Starting position: Place your hands on the prop, just a bit wider than shoulder-width apart. Step back with your feet just wider than shoulder-width to a distance that elongates your backside in a straight line from your heels to your head.

Action: Inhale as you slowly lower your body until your midchest is a few inches from the prop. Pause. Exhale as you press up, pulling your right arm up with you and bringing your wrist up to your lowest rib, allowing your elbow to brush by. Pause. Return your right hand to the ground as you inhale and lower your body. Repeat with the left arm. Alternate arms.

MODIFICATION

Harder: Perform on flat ground or inverted, with your feet propped up on a log or a bench.

FOCAL POINTS

- Think "wrist to ribs," keeping your wrist and elbow close to your low ribs as you pull.
- Keep your midchest in line with your hands.

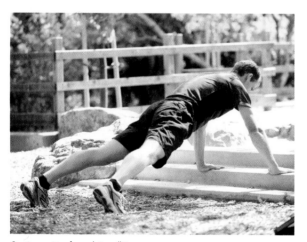

Starting position for push it–pull it

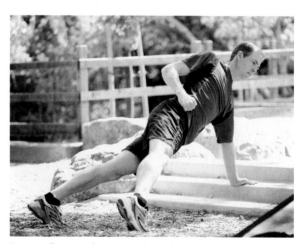

Press up pulling arm with you, wrist to lowest rib

Full-Body Press

Time is our most valuable commodity. Why just work the upper part of your body when, with the same amount of time and effort, you can include your lower body as well? Whatever your fitness level, it's my mission to make sure you get the most out of your time on the trail. This exercise targets your whole body quickly and effectively.

Works: Pectorals, deltoids, triceps, glutes, hamstrings, core stability.

Props: Flat terrain, step, log, bench, tabletop.

Starting position: Place your hands on the ground just a bit wider than shoulder-width apart. Step back to a distance that elongates your backside in a straight line from your heels to your head.

Action: Slowly lower your chest, while at the same time contracting your glutes as you lift your right leg at least 12 to 15 inches off the ground, flexing your right foot (point your toes toward your knee). Exhale up, pushing through your palms to lift your chest, while at the same time lowering your right leg. Alternate lifting your right and left legs.

MODIFICATIONS

Easier: Use a bench or the base of a staircase.

Harder: Perform on flat ground or inverted, with your feet propped up on a log or a bench.

FOCAL POINTS

- Maintain a hard flex to your foot as you lift it.
- Keep your midchest in line with your hands.
- Don't sag in the spine; instead, engage the abdominal wall for support.

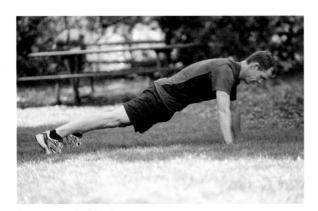

Starting position for full-body press

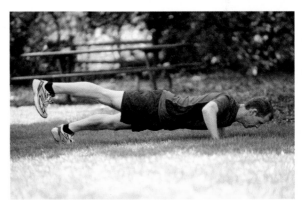

Lowering chest, lift leg with hard flex to foot

Full-Body Triceps Dip

I call this the "tri-it-you'll-like-it-dip"! Why work just your triceps when you can tone your entire body in the same amount of time? I created this exercise out of desperation. I was bored with the basic dip because it just didn't seem to be doing enough anymore. So I found a way to bring the full body into play, working abs, hamstrings, and glutes. All you need is a bench, curb, step, concrete block, low sea wall, log, boulder—or even the incline of a hill off a wooded trail.

Works: Triceps, deltoids, abdominals, hip flexors, quadriceps, hamstrings, glutes.

Props: Bench, log, low wall, step.

Starting position: From a seated position, place your hands hip-width apart, palms down and fingertips forward along the edge of the bench. Extend your legs in front of you, knees slightly bent and feet flexed against the ground.

Action: Lift your right leg, keeping it stick-straight, out in front of you. Begin to lower your body as you curl your right knee toward your chest to engage your abs. As you return to the starting position, press firmly through your palms and left heel to engage your triceps, as well as your glutes and hamstrings.

FOCAL POINTS

- Keep your tailbone very close to the prop as you lift and lower.
- I often see people sag around their neck and shoulders when they start to get fatigued. Don't sag—stay strong. Keep your shoulders down, away from your ears, by pressing firmly into the prop and lifting your chest up.

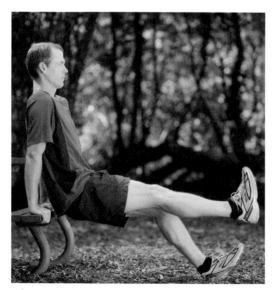

Starting position for full-body triceps dip

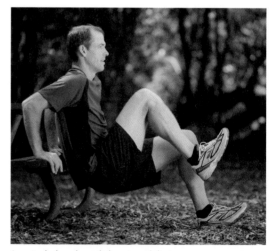

Lowering body, curling right knee toward chest

Rock-n-Balance

Balance is one of the most overlooked components of fitness. Did you know that in the United States, more than 300,000 people suffer broken hips every year? I came up with this exercise one fall day when I was training for ski season. I was bounding up a dry riverbed when I spotted a very pointy rock. I challenged myself to stand on the point for as long as I could. Later I added "foot scribing" exercises, such as spelling my name in huge loopy letters and trying to balance with my eyes closed.

This exercise can be done almost anywhere with a variety of props, including logs, tree roots, a parking curb, blocks,

> **TIP:** Don't be put off by wind. It will only enhance your practice and add a new dimension to your ability to use finesse, balance, mental focus, emotional power, and environmental integration training.

low-lying walls, or even a crimp in the sidewalk. The best prop is a stable, melon-size rock that protrudes out of the ground.

You'll especially enjoy this exercise because it allows you to interact with the elements. You'll have a completely different experience doing this exercise in the wind, rain, or fog than doing this exercise in sunshine, or while standing near

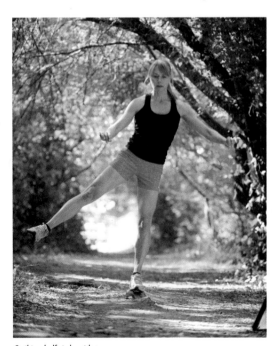

Starting position for rock-n-balance

Scribing half-circle with toes

a fountain or a waterfall. By exercising in different conditions, you enhance your skills as you become one with your surroundings—never fighting, only flowing.

Works: Hip flexors, abductors, ankles, glutes, balance, proprioceptive awareness, mental focus, emotional power, and environmental integration.

Props: Rock, root, curb.

Starting position: Find a stable rock, root, or bump protruding from the ground. Place the arch of your left foot on the pointiest or most rounded part of the rock—so that your foot and ankle may move in any range of motion. Find a focal point straight ahead, at least 20 feet away, and concentrate on it.

Action: Using your arms to help maintain balance, lift your opposite leg off the ground. Once you're feeling balanced, lift your leg higher and begin to scribe a half circle with your toes: forward, to the side, and behind you. Work from forward to back. And back to forward. Repeat with the other leg.

MODIFICATIONS

Easier: Stand on a flat surface and lift your right knee to hip height. Lower and tap the ground with your toes. Continue. Repeat with the other leg.

Your Core

Your core is your torso, the midsection of your body, including your abdominal muscles and the erector muscles of your lower back. But your core is much more than this—it is your body's foundation. You'll need a strong core for many things, including balance work. Core strength will be a priority in many of your workouts.

Harder:
- Increase time on each leg.
- Use the elements to your advantage—for example, a windy, rainy, or foggy day.
- Close your eyes.

FOCAL POINTS
- Gain stability through your center of mass.
- When you first do this exercise, you'll find you have one leg that is dominant or easier to balance on—over time, however, you'll find you can balance equally well on either leg.

Root Raise

Strengthen your shins and ankles with this simple, yet very effective exercise. The ever-changing terrain requires more work from your shins because you're continuously lifting and lowering your forefoot.

Works: Tibialis anterior (shins), ankle stability, balance.

Props: Step, tree root, curb, or parking block.

Starting position: From the athletic stance, place your heels on the prop, with your toes hanging over the side. Stand tall and keep your hands in your peripheral vision.

Action: Keeping your legs nearly straight, but not locked, lift and lower your toes, using full range of motion in your ankles. Avoid holding on to anything for balance.

FOCAL POINTS

For stability, imagine a large flashlight beaming light from your center of mass (below your navel) out into the distance at least 10 to 15 feet in front of you. Keep your eyes on the beam of light.

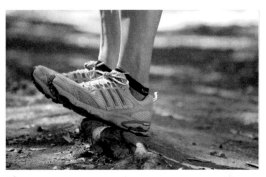

Lifting toes

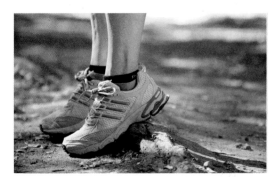

Lowering toes

TIP: There is something very primal, yet very soothing, about this exercise. On the one hand, you must feel the hard surface underfoot. To be successful, however, you must also be soft and flowing in your approach. Think too much about what you're doing, and you'll lose your balance.

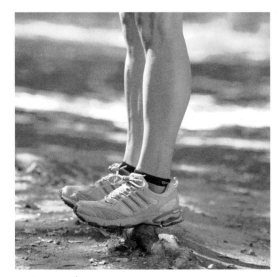

Starting position for root raise

TVA/March

By now you've learned how the simple TVA crunch can tone and flatten your abdominal wall. It's time to add to the intensity and results by incorporating this easy "march." The key to getting the most out of this move is by using finesse—feel every part of the movement and add extra focus to your deep abdominal muscles, which are doing the majority of the work, by pressing firmly into the ground.

Works: This version targets the deep stability muscles of the abdominals, plus a little on the sides.

Props: Flat surface—picnic table, bench, grass, sand, concrete.

Starting position: Use the same setup as the TVA crunch from your Base Moves (see chapter 5): Lie down on your back, knees bent, with your hands loosely behind your ears, elbows pointing to the sides, and your feet about 12 to 15 inches from your glutes.

> **TIP:** The key to this move is maintaining the pressure through your hips and tailbone.

Action: Press your hips and tailbone firmly into the ground—and maintain this pressure throughout the entire exercise. Now exhale up, lifting your right foot only a couple of inches off the ground, very slightly, as well as lifting your shoulder blades about an inch or 2 off the ground. Inhale as you slowly lower, placing (*not* plopping) your entire flat foot back down. Complete one set with your right foot, then repeat on the other side with your left foot. Or mix it up by alternating right and left.

FOCAL POINTS

- Throughout the exercise, press your lower abs firmly into your navel.
- Press your tailbone down, into the ground.

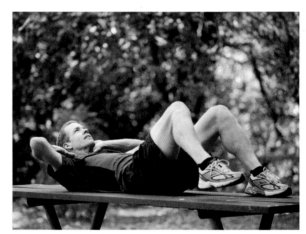

TVA/march—alternate lifting foot only a few inches

TVA/March "Harder"

Where this exercise is concerned, only the serious need apply! This is the ultimate "girdle" exercise, the one to strive for, especially because a little dose will do ya: 10 reps, and you're good to go.

Starting position: Set up the same way you would a regular TVA crunch, with your feet shoulder-width apart and as far away from your glutes as possible while maintaining a flat foot—big toe, little toe, and heel making contact.

Action: Press your hips and tailbone firmly into the ground—and maintain this pressure throughout the entire exercise. Exhale up, lifting both feet only a couple of inches off the ground (very slight), as well as lifting your shoulder blades about an inch or 2 off the ground. Inhale as you slowly lower—placing your entire flat foot back down.

FOCAL POINTS

Never allow your lower back to come off the ground. Use firm pressure to stabilize this area.

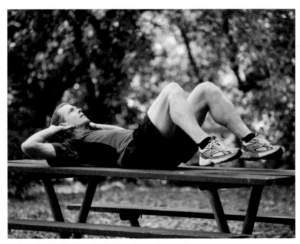

Make it harder by lifting both feet a few inches at the same time

Monkey-Bar Curl

Curls and crunches that emphasize the lower abdominal wall tend to be much more effective at tightening and toning. This monkey-bar curl does just that!

Works: Rectus abdominus (emphasis on the lower portion), hip flexors.

Props: Tree limb, monkey bar.

Starting position: Hang from a monkey bar, palms in an overhand grip.

Action: Exhale as you slowly lift your knees toward your chest. Inhale as you lower your knees as slowly as possible.

FOCAL POINTS

Don't swing your legs for momentum.

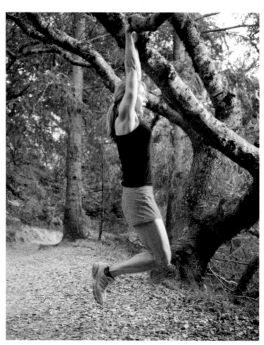

Starting position for monkey-bar curl

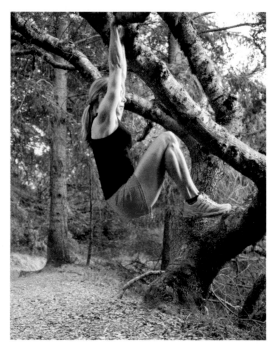

Lifting knees toward chest

Standing "C" Crunch

This exercise is designed to strengthen and tone your "six pack"—the strip of thick muscle from your lower ribs to your pelvis. The key to success is to make sure that you lengthen your abdominal wall completely by lengthening your arms overhead and your leg behind you, before you curl and contract ("crunch") it.

Works: Abdominal wall (rectus abdominus), hip flexors.

Props: Flat ground.

Starting position: Stand on flat ground, or if you're on a slight incline, face up the slope of the hill. From the athletic stance, turn your body to the left, at an angle. Lengthen your body by extending your arms overhead and your right leg slightly behind you, toes down, heel up.

TIP: The key here is finesse and using slight, yet powerful, controlled movement.

Action: Inhale as you lengthen your arms and leg enough to feel a stretch in your abdominal wall. Exhale as you pull your elbows down and lift your right knee up. Your elbows and knee pass each other as you curl and contract your abdominal wall, creating the letter C. Perform 12 to 25 repetitions, and then repeat with the other leg.

FOCAL POINTS

• Do your best to lay your body "out-and-over" the ground—think "table-top back" with eyes focused on the ground.

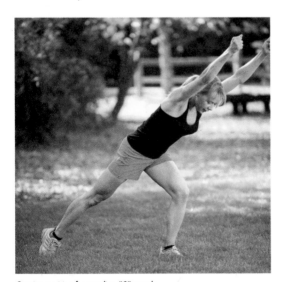

Starting position for standing "C" crunch

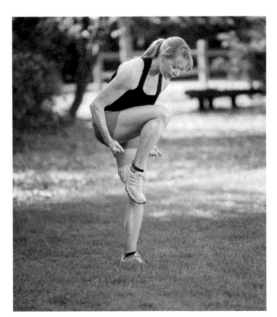

Curl and contract your abdominal wall to create the letter C

Standing Cross-Over Crunch

It's always good to mix it up and keep your body guessing. Change it up on your torso and shoulders with this cross-over crunch.

Works: Rectus abdominus, obliques, shoulders, hip flexors.

Props: Flat ground.

Starting position: With feet just beyond shoulder-width apart, activate your midsection by lifting your ribs up and away from your hips. Place your left hand on your hip for stability and so

you can feel the deep muscles of your core working. Hold your right arm in the goalpost position: elbow at shoulder height and bent at 90 degrees, palm facing forward in a fist.

Action: Lift your left knee toward your right shoulder, and at the same time cross your right elbow to meet your left knee. Your torso is creating the letter C, for *crunch.*

FOCAL POINTS

• Get the most out of the move by drawing your knee and elbow "out-and-away" from your body—and making contact.

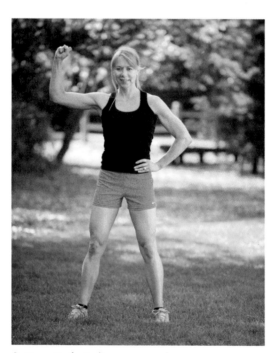

Starting position for standing cross-over crunch

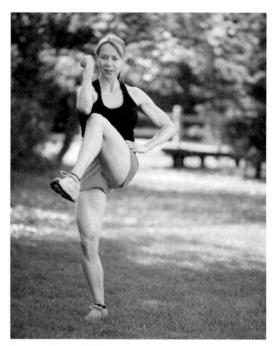

Knee and elbow meet in the center

Standing Oblique Crunch

My clients tell me they love this exercise because they can really feel the side of their waist getting "long and lean." The key is to *feel* every part of the movement, from reaching your arm over your head, to curling and contracting the side of your waist, with each and every repetition.

Works: Obliques, hips, shoulders.

Props: Flat ground.

Starting position: With feet just beyond shoulder-width apart, activate your midsection by lifting your ribs up and away from your hips. Place your left hand on your hip for stability and so you can feel the deep muscles of your core working. Extend your right arm over your head, with the palm facing forward and your hand balled up into a fist.

Action: Lift your right knee laterally, while at the same time pulling your elbow down to meet your right knee. Your side is creating the letter C, for *crunch.*

FOCAL POINTS

• Keep in mind that in order to change a muscle, it must go through the *eccentric,* or stretching phase, before the *concentric,* or contracting phase; so reach up to the sky and feel your side lengthen before you go into the crunch.

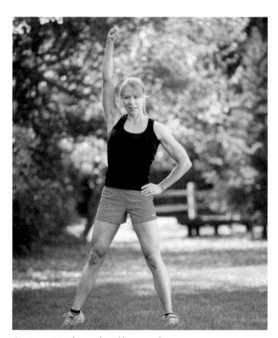

Starting position for standing oblique crunch

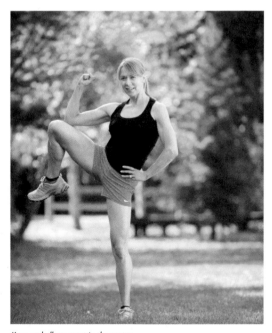

Knee and elbow meet in the center

Aqua Pulse

It's not enough to do abdominal work; you also need to work the opposing muscle group—your lower back, or erectors. This will support your spine, improve posture, and prevent back injuries. Aqua and aqua-type exercises, which work this muscle group, are perfect to do on the beach while you listen to the crashing of the waves.

Works: Backside and erectors (the muscles that line the spine).

Props: Flat surface—picnic table, bench, grass, sand, concrete.

Starting position: Set up the same way you do for the Base Move aqua (see chapter 5): Lie face down on the ground with your head in line with your spine.

Lengthen your arms out long overhead, palms down on the ground.

Actions: Lift your right arm and left leg. Lift and lower your arm and leg with a small controlled movement that feels like pulsing (without touching the ground), lifting up and down about 1 to 2 inches. Start with 15 reps per side, then 10 per side, and end with 5 per side.

MODIFICATION

Harder: Start with 25 to 30 per side, then subtract 5 with each set until you reach 5 per side.

FOCAL POINTS

• Keep your body long—imagine there is someone pulling on your fingertips as well as your toes.

TIP: Technically, abdominal and core work can be done every day. However, to prevent injuries, always do them at the *end* of your workout. Your abs and core are your stabilizers, and you don't want to burn them out before you're done. To keep your routine fresh and your abs responding, mix it up! Add twisting and rotating work to sculpt your waist.

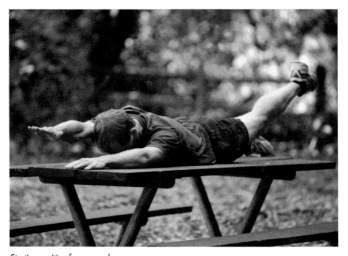

Starting position for aqua pulse

Workout 4:
Single Site—
Steps and Stairs

WORKOUT SNAPSHOT

Total time: 45 to 60 minutes.
Props: Steps, stairs, bleachers.
Location: High school athletic field, park, or plaza—just so long as it has steps.
Purpose: Cardio, muscular strength and endurance, balance and agility, full body and core strength, multidirectional movement.

I love step and stair workouts! This workout puts any gym routine to shame. You're constantly keeping your body guessing and your mind focused. It's also a favorite of mine because it's the kind of session you can take anywhere, even when you're traveling. You can find a set of bleachers, or a long set of steps, in nearly any city or country setting.

Working on stairs is a blast, but it does require some extra attention to safety. Incorporate these guidelines for stair work to make sure you have a safe and effective session:

• Use only the muscles you need for the climb or descent, and relax the ones you don't.

• Maintain a soft eye focus, which lets you read your terrain peripherally.

• Stay mindfully connected to your feet—a sense of the texture underfoot will prevent injury and let you move gracefully and efficiently.

• Use metaphors for inspiration and for fun. Tell yourself: "Move like a gazelle, not an elephant!" Think: "Bunny feet, not elephant feet."

• Be cautious and aware of the conditions: icy, wet, slippery surfaces; worn wood; wet leaves and twigs; gravel and sand.

Relax Your Resting Muscles

Muscles are either on or off. There is no in between—either your muscles are firing and contracted, using energy, or they are not. There's no such thing as "kind of contracted." Get to know your muscles, and pay attention to what muscles you need when. If you're familiar with the muscles your body is using, you can relax the muscles you're not using. No more white-knuckling, folks!

Use these safety strategies when descending the stairs:

- Keep your hands within your peripheral vision—*never* in your pockets.
- To prevent spills, especially on wet surfaces, use the toe-heel technique. First lower your foot onto the step, tapping your toes and the ball of your foot on the surface. Then lightly snap your heel into the pocket of the step. As long as your heel makes contact with the surface, you will not stumble.
- Finesse is important. To prevent slipping, make sure you don't place too much pressure under the ball of your foot.
- Move straight down the steps and not across them.

Stage 1: Warm-Up (10 minutes)

Warm-Up Walk (5 minutes)

Before you get into your warm-up exercises, take a 3- to 5-minute walk around your site. Include a couple of trips up and down the steps, stairs, or bleachers. You are warming up your body, and you're also getting both your body and mind used to the new terrain, including the height and texture of the steps. Take it slow, and make sure you hit every step with great form and posture.

After your warm-up walk, do the following warm-up exercises on the bottom step.

1. High knees—2 sets of 10 to 20 reps per leg. (See chapter 4.)
2. Kickbacks—2 sets of 10 to 20 reps.

Next you'll continue your warm-up moving up the steps. Put your hands on your hips, with your fingertips touching your abdominal wall. Take a step up and contract your glutes, extending your leg behind you. Do your best to place your full foot up onto the step, and as you rise, press your heel firmly into the step as you lift your leg. Perform 10 to 20 reps, counting "1, 2, 3 . . ." as you alternate your legs moving up the steps.

Walk normally for 10 to 20 steps and resume with another set of 10 to 20 reps. Continue this pattern to the top of the stairs, and then head back down for a full recovery.

To wrap up your warm-up, take a moment to stretch your hip flexors, hamstrings, quadriceps, inner thighs, and calves.

> **TIP:** Prevent lower-back strain when ascending steps or stairs by tilting forward at the hips in a straight line with your back foot. Maintain a strong abdominal wall for support.

Go Slow to Go Fast!

So often I see people jump from their cars right into a run. This is bad for both body and mind. If you fling yourself directly into a run, your heart rate jumps very high, very fast. This will put you immediately in an anaerobic state. Your body will start producing lactic acid, your legs will become stiff, and you'll feel a burning sensation in your muscles and joints. It's easy to get discouraged when you're winded and in pain right at the start of your workout.

Instead, go slow to go fast. Take the time to get your entire engine "lubed up." This includes your muscles, your joints, and your mind. A proper warm-up puts you in control, makes you strong, and keeps you relaxed.

Stage 2: Muscular Strength and Endurance Exercises

For each exercise do 2 sets of 10 to 20 reps. Do the first 2 exercises at the base of the steps.

"Half-Tuck" Squat

This is a great exercise for your legs, especially the inner thighs. Just make sure that you press firmly through the arch of your foot with each lift.

MODIFICATIONS

Easier: Lower your hips only 1 to 2 inches before pressing back up to the starting position.

Harder: Hold the position for 2 to 3 counts before pressing back up to the starting position.

"Push It–Pull It"

The stability of your core muscles comes into play with this exercise, which activates both the pushing muscles of your chest and the pulling muscles of your back.

MODIFICATIONS

Easier: Take a higher position on the stairs so you are at a greater incline.

Harder: Invert this exercise, with your feet on the steps and your hands flat on the ground. Pause for 1 to 3 counts at the bottom of the move before pushing pack up.

Cardio Blast
(2 to 3 minutes; RPE 8)

Let 'er rip! You'll spike your metabolism with several rounds on the stairs to get your heart rate up and blast some calories. Take off slowly. Gradually build your RPE to 8 by pumping your arms to set your tempo. Work on your quickness and agility by hitting every step on the way up and the way down. Use the down trips to recover completely.

> **TIP:** To protect your lower back, keep your back straight and lean into the incline of the slope from your hips.

Lateral Press

This is a fun twist on the lateral press—it's sort of a cross between the lateral press and a sumo because you travel up the steps sideways with your hips low and your knees bent at about 45 degrees.

MODIFICATIONS

Easier: Take a shorter stride and lower your tailbone no more than an inch.
Harder: Squat down lower and move slower. Never allow your tailbone to raise and lower during the exercise. Remember, the lower your tailbone, the more challenging the move. So work your way "down" over time.

Step Lunges

Use the same technique as you do for walking and traveling lunges, but place an even greater emphasis on control of the movement, especially over loose and wet terrain.

MODIFICATIONS

Easier: Take a shorter stride, only lowering your hips about 1 to 2 inches.
Harder: Pause for a count and exhale as you press firmly through your back toes, moving yourself to the next step.

Cardio Blast
(2 to 3 minutes; RPE 8–9)

Take off slowly. Gradually build your RPE to 8 or 9. Use the down trips to recover completely.

> **TIP:** As you climb hills and stairs, it's important to control your breathing. Breathe low and slow, and don't let your breathing control you. This leads to gasping, slowing down, feeling ill, and going anaerobic. Breathing is a health and fitness tool. When you learn how to use your breathing to your advantage, your workouts will become easier and less stressed.

Sumo Squat

This exercise can get intense pretty quickly! Your heart rate will climb as you do these. Just remember to breathe "low and slow," exhaling on the exertion part of the movement.

MODIFICATIONS

Easier: Take a shorter stride, only lowering your hips about 1 to 2 inches.

Harder: Lower until your knees create a 90-degree angle, and then add a lateral leg lift with each step up.

Diagonal Stride

Get low and lean into the hill, like a skater, using your glutes and legs for this powerful exercise. Don't let momentum do the work here.

TIP: Save energy and experience a more successful climb with a technique I call double stepping. Develop a rhythm by lightly tapping both feet on the step in a left-right or right-left pattern. This encourages consistency and will help to ease burning legs. By alternating your foot-climbing pattern, your legs will relax more and receive more oxygenated blood.

MODIFICATION

Harder: As you lift, move more quickly, brushing the lifted knee and ankle just past the support leg.

No Venous Pooling

When you reach the top of a long set of stairs, or a steep hill, it's tempting to stop and try to catch your breath. Don't do this! Stopping suddenly after a strenuous climb can lead to what's called venous pooling, which occurs when blood collects in the limbs. When you push your body to exert itself, your heart rate naturally climbs in order to pump more blood and oxygen to the working muscles. If you stop suddenly, your heart is still pumping rapidly. All of that blood has to go somewhere, and so it pools in your limbs. Venous pooling, especially in the legs, creates pressure and can cause broken capillaries and lead to varicose veins. Rather than stopping cold at the top of an incline, keep your legs moving. Walk it out while you catch your breath.

Cardio Blast
(2 to 3 minutes; RPE 8–9)

Last one! Give it what you've got, working on your quickness and agility by hitting every step on the way up and the way down. Walk it out for a few minutes before moving on to calf raises.

MODIFICATION

Easier: Build your RPE to 7 or 7.5, which keeps you working aerobically (with oxygen).

Calf Raise

See chapter 5 for a description of the calf raise, but do it this time three different ways: toes straight, toes in, and toes out!

Stage 3: Cooldown (10 minutes)

TVA/Ab Flattener (2 sets)

See chapter 5 for a description of this exercise. Recover for 20 seconds before performing your second set. Maintain even pressure between your navel and your pelvis the entire time.

Aqua (2 sets)

See chapter 5 for a description of this exercise. After your first set, take 30 seconds to recover and relax your back. You can pull your hips back and over your feet to give your back a stretch. For your second set, try aqua pulse.

Flexibility

On a flat spot, lie on your back and pull your knees up to your chest. Take a deep breath. As you exhale, pull your knees more closely to your chest as you relax and release your lower back. With each exhalation, relax your body and sink more deeply into the surface below you. Take this opportunity to go to the core of your core: quiet your mind and just be.

Recommended Stretches

See chapter 4.
- Hip flexors
- Hamstrings
- Quadriceps
- Inner thighs (adductors)
- Calves

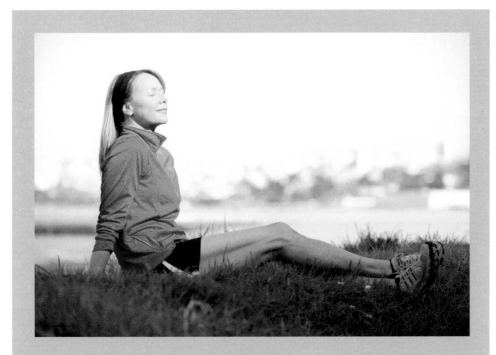

Thanksuary: The Core of Your Core

My hope for you is that each and every session is an adventure and an experience that is both invigorating and peaceful. With a little scouting, you'll find many places where you can stimulate your body, draw power from your surroundings, and center and quiet your mind. You will enjoy not just a full-body experience, but a *full-being* experience: body, mind, and soul.

I have found special quiet places in my neighborhood where I've connected deeply at various times, and whenever I return I can instantly get to that place: the "core of my core." It's a combination of familiarity, sensory affiliation, and emotional conditioning that takes me there. I call these special places my "Thanksuary"—places where I experience a deep feeling of gratitude. I've learned that feelings of thankfulness and gratitude are actually stress reducers. While you're engaged in feeling grateful, it is difficult—if not impossible—for your BodyMind to experience stress and anxiety. In your cooldown today, and on any day when you are moved to, find your own Thanksuary.

Workout 5: Multisite— Urban Neighborhood or Downtown Plaza

WORKOUT SNAPSHOT

Total time: 45 to 60 minutes.

Props: Parking meter or pole, low wall or bench, curb or parking stop.

Location: Urban neighborhood or downtown plaza.

Purpose: Muscular strength and endurance, cardio, full-body and core strength, multidirectional movement, balance and agility, proprioceptive awareness, kinesthetic awareness, mental focus.

It may come as a surprise, but urban areas can be inspiring places to exercise, full of challenges and stimulation. The best time to do an urban or downtown workout is in the early morning. The air is fresh, the streets are quiet, and you will feel as though you have the whole city to yourself.

The props you'll need for this multi-site workout are things you'll find in any small or large city: a parking meter or a pole such as a stop sign; a bench or a low wall; a curb or a low parking stop. You can rearrange the sequence of the strength exercises to make them fit with your particular environment and the order in which you find your props. Also, keep in mind that the workout moves from station to station, so each exercise falls under a particular station or site.

Stage 1: Warm-Up (5 to 10 minutes)

By now you've learned what works best for you in your warm-up. Whatever you do, just don't skip it. This warming-up time is as important as the workout itself. See chapter 4 for full descriptions of these moves.

1. Joint lubrication
2. Reverse breath
3. Cardio walk or run to station 1 (RPE 6)

Continue to warm up with a fast walk or a slow jog for 5 to 10 minutes, gradually bringing your RPE to 6, a low aerobic level. Take a moment to stretch your hip flexors, hamstrings, quadriceps, and calves—anything that may feel tight.

Stage 2: Exercises (30 to 40 minutes)

Perform each exercise for 60 seconds (or 30 seconds per side).

Station 1—Flat Ground

Wide-Legged Squat with Overhead Reach

See chapter 5. It's easy to achieve a "two-for-one" by incorporating your upper and lower body into one exercise. As you squat down, reach your arms overhead and inhale. As you stand up, pull your elbows down at a 90-degree angle, at shoulder height, in a "goalpost" position. Feel your chest open as you pull your shoulder blades together. Remember to inhale as you lower and exhale as you stand.

TIP: Observe how your lungs open up when you reach overhead and inhale at the same time.

MODIFICATIONS

Easier: Lower your hips only a couple of inches.

Harder: Bend your knees to a 90-degree angle and pause at the bottom of the move for 1 to 3 counts before returning to your starting position.

Forward-to-Reverse Lunge

See chapter 5. Begin by doing a forward lunge, followed by a reverse lunge.

TIP: Contract the glutes of the standing or "support" leg as you move forward to reverse in these lunges. This will take some of the fatigue out of the exercise.

MODIFICATIONS

Easier: Alternate between the right and left side rather than doing all your reps on the same side.

Harder: Add an isometric bicep curl to the forward lunge and an isometric upright row to the reverse lunge.

Cardio Travel
(2 to 3 minutes, RPE 7–7.5)

Take it sideways as you steadily build your heart rate. Use the lines on the sidewalks as a guide to keep your feet in a linear position so you can press firmly through the arch of your foot.

Lateral "Line" Press

See the lateral leg press Base Move in chapter 5.) Engage that core; keep your palms up and your arms lifted the entire time. Keep your RPE at 7 to 7.5.

Switch legs and perform another series of lateral presses, leading with the other leg, for 30 to 60 seconds. Engage your core throughout this exercise by maintaining good posture.

Walk it out for 30 seconds and move to your next station.

Station 2— Parking Meter or Pole

Parking Meter Press
High and tight!

Full-Body Lunge

MODIFICATIONS
Easier: Perform these lunges with a long step. Lower your hips only about 1 to 2 inches and hold your arms out laterally, at shoulder height.

Harder: Bend your forward knee to 90 degrees.

Safety tips for lunges:
- Perform each lunge in a controlled manner—slower is better.
- Maintain tight abdominals to support your lumbar spine and knees.
- Prevent lower-back strain—especially on hills and steps—by tilting forward slightly from the hips.

- Distribute your weight evenly between both feet.
- Do not let your knee extend beyond your shoelaces.
- Focus your gaze at least 10 to 15 feet ahead.
- Exhale during the "up," or exertion, phase.

Cardio: Lateral Sidewalk Shuffle (2 to 3 minutes; RPE 7–7.5)

This is similar to the lateral leg press, but this time you're going to fire it up a notch!

Take off, moving sideways along the sidewalk. Lower your hips and press your palms firmly together, keeping them in line with your sternum. Begin by taking a wide step onto your right foot. Keeping your hips low and your back straight, press through the arch of your left foot, from big toe to heel. As you move quickly along the sidewalk, think "step, feet together, step, feet together." Continue for 30 to 60 seconds, with your

---

Lunges

Lunges are probably the most effective lower-body exercise around. They strengthen and tone your legs, hips, and glutes. When you add an upper-body move like an upright row or overhead press, you also work your core. What's more, every time you do a set of lunges, your heart rate will land smack-dab in the middle of *your* aerobic zone. Every time!

RPE at 7 to 7.5. Repeat for another 30 to 60 seconds, leading with the other leg.

Station 3— Bench or Low Wall

Full-Body Triceps Dip

MODIFICATIONS

Easier: March in place by lifting one knee up as you dip down, and then the other knee up as you dip down.

Harder: Move in slow motion. Dip down slowly, hold for a count, and slowly exhale up.

Full-Body Press

MODIFICATIONS

Easier: Use a greater incline by working with a table, a mailbox, or a wall.

Harder: Use flat terrain and perform each repetition in slow motion, pausing at the bottom of the move.

Cardio: "Walk the Line" (2 to 3 minutes); RPE 7–7.5

Find a line in the sidewalk, a raised curb, or a line along the curb. Run or walk as quickly as you can along the curb, placing one foot directly in front of the other. Focus on your form and foot placement. Use your hands for counterbalance and lower your hips to keep a quick, even pace.

Walk it out until your RPE comes down to a 3. As you're walking, scout out a spot for the next exercise—a crimp in the sidewalk, a parking block, an embedded rock, or a root in the grass.

Station 4— Curb or Step

Calf Raise

See chapter 5.
Repeat Stage 2 circuit (optional).

Stage 3: Cooldown (5 to 10 minutes)

Cardio Cooldown (RPE 5)

Almost done! Head back to your start, holding at an RPE of 5. Use your low and slow breathing to wash your body with oxygen and clear out any lactic acid. Also, use this segment to clear your body and mind of any tension.

PMJ Exercise

Remember how most of our thoughts come in three types: plans, memories, and judgments. Referring to chapter 2, use this mindfulness exercise while you're out on the path to clear your mind, root out the cobwebs, and let go of any lingering tension or stress.

Flexibility (5 minutes)

Workout 6: Traveling— Rural Park or Path

WORKOUT SNAPSHOT
Total time: 45 to 60 minutes.
Props: Tree or wall.
Location: A 1- to 5-mile loop or path that contains hills.
Purpose: Cardio, muscular strength and endurance, full-body and core strength, balance and agility, multidirectional movement.

Flexibility (5 minutes)

This is a wonderful traveling workout that can be adapted to any number of environments. The workout calls for a couple of stops at hillsides, but if your best location is a riverside path, or another location without inclines, just do these exercises on flat ground. The same thing goes for tree sits. If you're in an open field, or another place without sturdy trees nearby, use a telephone pole or a wall.

When you're planning a traveling workout, ideally you want to choose a path that has as much variety as possible, with different types of terrain and access to different prop structures. As you get familiar with the individual exercises and the sequence of the workouts, you'll become even more adept at choosing locations that work best for you and your goals.

Stage 1: Warm-Up (5 to 10 minutes)

See chapter 4 for descriptions of these moves.

1. Joint lubrication
2. Reverse breath
3. Cardio: fairly quick walk or easy run

This easy warm-up walk or jog should take your RPE to a level 4 or 5, which is a moderate effort. Use your arm swing to set your tempo. As you build speed, be sure to read and record your terrain. Look 10 to 15 feet ahead of you and scan the path for any lumps, bumps, twists, or turns.

Stage 2: Location Exercises

Station 1— Hillside

Hill Squat (1 minute)

These are my favorite squats on the planet. A hillside can actually provide a stable and effective platform for working your glutes and hamstrings—especially the area where the two meet.

TIP: The more firmly you press through your heels, the more you'll work your glutes and hamstrings!

Reach Out and Touch Something

You've grown accustomed to smelling the fresh air and taking in all the colorful sights during your workout. Now it's time to touch nature. When was the last time you ran your hand across a tree limb or stuck your nose in a flower? Make time for moments in your workout when you can make direct physical contact with the natural world around you. It will only deepen the connection you're establishing with your environment.

Cardio Travel
(3 minutes; RPE 6–7)

During this run, build your RPE to a 6 or 7. Feel the earth through your feet. Remember to breathe low and slow. Stay relaxed as your heart rate rises.

When you come to the 2½-minute mark, scout around for a tree, post, or wall for sits. As you near the spot, bring your run down to a walk for about 30 seconds, until your RPE is about 3.

Station 2—
Tree

Tree Sit (1 minute)

These sits work your quads—hard! They also engage your deep core muscles, your hip flexors, and your shoulders, as well as challenge your balance and mental focus.

Tree Stand—Lower Body
(30 to 60 seconds per side)

This exercise works your hamstrings, glutes, core stability, shoulders, and balance.

Cardio Travel (3 minutes; RPE 7)

Walk for 30 seconds or so before you start jogging to your next station. You're in the full flow of your workout now, so in this cardio session build to an RPE of 7. Go with the flow as you run. Feel gravity holding your body. Don't fight anything—just flow.

At 2½ minutes, look for a tree, a set of monkey bars, or a low fence for your next two exercises. You need a tree with a strong base and a limb low enough to grasp. Slow to a walk and bring your RPE to 3 or 4.

Station 3—
Tree or Fence

One-Armed Press
(30 to 60 seconds per side)

This is a powerful arm, chest, and shoulder strengthener. When you are finished, take an "active recovery" break and walk it out for 30 seconds before moving on to the next exercise.

"Palm-to-Palm" Pull-Up (1 minute)

This exercise works your upper back, shoulders, and biceps. Select a prop—a tree limb or a monkey bar—that is just above the height of your head. Many people feel they simply can't do a pull-up. Not anymore! This is a much easier version of the classic pull-up. And once you've finished with the serious work of the exercise, it's time for some monkey business! Hanging from a tree is a fun, childlike way to stretch out your back.

Cardio Travel
(3 minutes; RPE 7–8)

You're deep into your workout, so bring your RPE to 7 or even 8 for this next cardio block. Observe how much easier and more pleasurable it is to exercise when you are integrated with your environment. Take a moment to picture yourself moving with the power and grace of a gazelle—or some other sleek, graceful, and dynamic animal.

At 2½ minutes, be on the lookout for an incline or a hill for your next two exercises. Walk for 30 seconds.

Station 4—
Hillside

Remember to perform the next two exercises as you travel *up* the hill.

Diagonal Stride
(1 to 2 minutes)

"The redwoods have got your back"

My friends and I have a saying: "The redwoods have got your back." When one of us is feeling stressed, is working through a problem, or is simply feeling out of sorts, we go into the forest for fresh air, exercise, and solitude, which helps us to work through the difficulty. Sometimes when you're "in it," it's tough to see the forest through the trees and remember the many gifts nature has to offer—clarity, serenity, peace, and inspiration—so we'll use this one phrase as a reminder. We head for the forest. That's all it takes. And remember, the redwoods have your back.

Uneven Terrain Makes You Stronger—and Smaller!

Another reason to love these outdoor exercises is that you are constantly working in all planes of motion over uneven terrain, which causes the deep layers of your core, known as the inner unit, to fire and work. When you work these deeper layers, your abs, waist, and lower back not only get stronger, they get smaller.

MODIFICATION

Harder: As you lift, move more quickly, brushing the lifted knee and ankle past the support leg.

Sumo Squat
(1 to 2 minutes per side)

This exercise is extremely effective for sculpting the inner and outer thighs, as well as the hips and glutes. Walk it out for 30 seconds before moving on to the next station.

Cardio Travel
(3 minutes; RPE 6–7)

Use this cardio block to clear your mind and body of tension. Take your RPE to a 6 or 7. Focus on maintaining strong posture: chest open, chin up, eyes forward. Use a nice even arm swing to maintain your tempo. Even breathing is critical in this stage of your workout, in order to wash your body with oxygen and clear out any lactic acid that has built up in your system. After 3 minutes, walk it out for 30 seconds.

Station 5— Flat Ground

You've accomplished a lot in about 30 minutes, focusing on both your upper and lower body. Now it's time to work on your core strength. Keeping with the theme of this workout, you'll get a lot done in a little time. Working your midsection while standing up will help you use more muscle fiber in your deep abdominal muscles.

Standing "C" Crunch
(1 minute—30 to 60 seconds per side)

The standing curl targets not only the deep layers of the abdominal wall, it challenges your hip flexors, glutes, heart, and lungs.

TIP: Lift your knee out and away from your body and then up to your chest, so that you form the letter C. For support and stability, contract your glutes in the support leg. Repeat on the other side.

Standing Cross-Over Crunch
(1 minute—30 seconds per side)

This crunch works your obliques, hips, and shoulders. After you're through, walk it out for 30 seconds to catch your breath and clear your mind. Draw in a few deep breaths and exhale completely.

Stage 3:
Cardio and Cooldown
(5 to 20 minutes)

Remember, your cooldown is just as important as your warm-up. You will gradually lower your heart rate, prevent venous pooling in your limbs, clear out lactic acid, prevent muscle cramping and stiffness, and regulate your cardiac rhythm.

> **TIP:** Close your eyes and allow your olfactory sense to take the lead. What do you smell? Did it rain last night? Has the grass been cut recently?

Cardio Walk or Jog Back to Start
(5 to 10 minutes)

Use the HeartBrain technique as a mental exercise during this cooldown. To review this technique, remember that your heart has a mind of its own—those amazing cells and neurotransmitters that together can learn, remember, and respond independently of the brain. When you lead with your heart, you make a deep connection to your inner self and to your environment. Here's a HeartBrain meditative walk (or jog) that lets you "follow your heart" in a moving meditation:

1. Stand tall with your eyes closed. Breathe in, following the flow of air deeply into your chest and belly. Continue to observe this flowing of breath as you relax your mind. Just be. Remain focused on your chest until you feel solidly connected to your heart.

2. When you feel connected, open your eyes.

3. Focus your eyes about 10 to 15 feet in front of you and begin to walk as you continue to breathe and maintain that heart connection. From a strong, erect posture, imagine your heart and chest leading you along the path. Maintain a soft eye focus, where all you notice are colors and textures in your vision. (Some call this "Buddha's eyes.")

4. Slowly bump up your pace to either a quick walk or a gentle jog to your starting place. Keep your soft eye focus, breathe deeply, and let your heart lead you.

Rock in Your Pocket

Toward the end of a group workout and before moving into a cardio cooldown, I often suggest to my clients that they pick up an attractive rock or stone to hold in their hand. At that point, we'll take a few minutes to find a quiet place to sit, meditate, and focus on a goal, wish, or happy thought for the day. As each member becomes absolutely clear and centered, she will take off on her 5- to 10-minute cooldown, all the while holding the rock and focusing on her goal or happy thought. Then, after the workout is done, and throughout the rest of the day, she'll keep the rock in her pocket and reach for it anytime she needs a happy reminder of the peace she had achieved earlier in the day.

5. If you lose focus, simply start again. Relax, take deep breaths, connect to your chest and heart, and follow your heart back.

Flexibility

Once you reach your starting point, walk until your RPE is 2 to 3 before you begin a full body stretch, including the following (see chapter 4):

- Hip flexors
- Hamstrings
- Quadriceps
- Calves
- Inner thighs (adductors)
- Chest, shoulders, and biceps
- Back
- Upper back and rear shoulders

CHAPTER 7

Phase 3: Sustenance, Weeks 9 through 12 and Beyond

You've arrived at the future of your fitness life! Phase 3 is all about sustaining and experiencing great joy and satisfaction as you maintain your level of health and fitness for the rest of your life. You will need to continue to make adaptations—to keep feeding surprises to your body and mind, and just to keep things fun for yourself. When you reach this stage, not only will you miss exercise when you miss a workout, but both your body and mind will need to work out to feel good. You're at a place where fitness feels like "I get to!" instead of "I have to!"

In this phase, you'll meet your goals and set new ones. You'll take your body's health and physical prowess to new levels, sharpen your mental focus and acuity to reach new performance heights, and experience the great freedom that true BodyMind fitness and health bring as you:

- Increase your cardiovascular health and fat-burning ability
- Increase your body's ability to build and maintain muscle mass
- Increase and hold on to bone density
- Strengthen your body's immune system and ability to fight illness
- Train for sports performance
- Own the ability to enhance/change your mood/emotional outlook in an instant

One of the keys to the program that we've learned is that discipline, willpower, and control don't work. Essentially, we aren't moved by thinking or willing it to happen—we are not driven by logical thought. We know now that *emotions* drive us—we do things to our detriment or benefit when driven by our emotions. Nature is a powerful source in our emotional, physical, and mental health and well-being.

The workouts in Phase 3 help set you up to continue your Outdoor Fitness practice long after you've reached the 12-week point. Workout 7 lets you be a kid again with a circuit training session at your local playground or park. This workout delivers a full-body muscular strength session that you can customize to your time constraints as well as your environment. Workout 8 is another any-time, anywhere session that emphasizes core and cardio training while putting your body through moves that challenge your range of motion. Workout 9 really kicks things up a notch, introducing you to a powerful new aspect in your fitness arsenal: interval training. Speed, agility, and quickness (SAQ) are the keys to this session, which is based on speed drills that help you blast fat and boost your metabolism while you strengthen your muscles and cardiovascular system.

Workout 7:
Single Site—Playground

WORKOUT SNAPSHOT
Total time: 30 to 60 minutes.
Props: Pole or post, tree limb or bar, base of tree or wall, sand or grass.
Location: Playground.
Purpose: Total body muscular strength.

This single-site workout is a simple strength-training circuit that uses the props and terrain found in most play-grounds. This is an easy-to-adapt ses-sion, the kind of workout that you can slip in while still keeping an eye on your kids at the playground. You'll work your full body in these muscular strength exer-cises so efficiently that you'll be finished before your kids start bugging you about what's for lunch.

Stage 1:
Warm-Up
(5 to 10 minutes)

If you are doing a "one-spot warm-up," follow the routine below at your loca-tion. If you're able to include a walk to your site, then combine your cardio with joint rotations and breathing. (For descriptions of these warm-up exercises, see chapter 4.)

1. Joint lubrication (1 minute)
2. Reverse breath and posture check (1 minute)
3. Cardio warm-up (3-5 minutes)
   - High knees (1 minute)
   - Step-ups (1-2 minutes)
   - Lateral step-ups (1-2 minutes)

Remember, form and alignment are as important to exercise as the movements themselves. Paying attention to your posture, and keeping your body aligned, keeps you safe from injury, makes your movements more efficient and powerful, and helps your "body intelligence." Over time, as you stick to great form and posture, your body will learn the feeling of alignment and will fall into form more easily and naturally.

Stage 2: Total Body Muscular Strength Circuit (20 to 30 minutes)

These exercises represent Base Moves as well as Signature Moves, which are described in more detail in chapters 5 and 6, respectively. Perform 12 to 20 reps for each exercise, depending on your time constraints and fitness level. Pay attention to keeping good form throughout each set. If you find that you're unable to get through an entire set without breaking form, move into the "easier" modification or take a breather and continue with the exercise when you can maintain your form. Once you've completed the entire circuit, go back and repeat it a second time.

Wide-Legged Squats with "Palm-to-Palm" Press

MODIFICATIONS

Easier: Lower your hips only a couple of inches.

Harder: Bend your knees to a 90-degree angle and pause at the bottom of the move for 1 to 3 counts before returning to your starting position.

One-Armed Press

This is a great exercise to build strength in your arms, chest, and shoulders. Remember to take an "active recovery" break and walk it out for 30 seconds before moving on to the next exercise.

Parking Meter Press

If you're feeling tight, be sure to stretch out your hamstrings and your glutes before moving on to the next exercise.

Tree Sit

Plant it here for killer quads! You'll also work your deep core muscles, and your shoulders. To prevent slipping, clear away gravel, twigs, and debris from underfoot.

MODIFICATION

Harder: March in place, lifting your foot only a few inches off the ground.

"Palm-to-Palm" Pull-Up

MODIFICATION

Easier: Place one foot against the tree or bar for leverage.

Full-Body Press

MODIFICATIONS

Easier: Use more of an incline, from a wall, a table, or a mailbox.

Harder: Use flat terrain and perform each repetition in slow motion, pausing at the bottom of the move.

TIP: Just because you're in the middle of a playground and not in the middle of the woods doesn't mean you can't practice your environmental integration. Open up your senses. Do you hear kids laughing? What does the ground feel like beneath your feet?

Tree Stand—Lower Body

This is a great core stability strengthener that allows you to reach out and touch a tree.

Tree Stand—Upper Body

This is an excellent exercise to build balance and mental focus.

Review: Concentration, Intensity, and Relaxation

Remember the keys to athletic success? They are concentration, intensity, and relaxation. You need the ability to focus on your task at hand, blocking out the psychological static that so often plagues all of us; to be able to perform while fully absorbed in the moment; and to be able to let go of tension.

When you relax, the world slows down around you. You've heard about being "in the zone." This is a component of entering that zone. When you are tense, you use up precious energy tightening your muscles and getting stuck "in your head." Relaxation is a skill that has to be developed, just like concentration and intensity. Think to yourself:

Be a kid!
Play with the terrain!
Stay loose!
Go with the flow!

Tree Hang or Monkey Bar Hang

Most of us are stuck sitting at a desk all day. When we're not at our desks, we're sitting in the car, on the bus, or in our living rooms. All this sitting leaves you with compressed and restricted muscles and joints, especially in your back, shoulders, and hips. You can release the kinks and tension and also feel close to nature and your childlike self with this easy and fun exercise: Simply hang from a tree limb or bar. As you hang, take a deep breath in, and then completely exhale. As you exhale, relax your body, especially your hips and pelvis. You will feel your spine begin to lengthen.

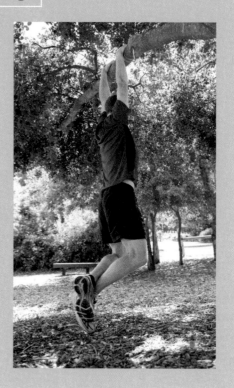

Standing Oblique Crunch

This exercise focuses on your hips and shoulders as well as your obliques.

Monkey-Bar Curl

Focus on performing the exercise using your abdominals to do the work. Avoid swinging your legs for momentum.

Stage 3:
Cooldown and Flexibility (5 to 10 minutes)

Perform your regular cooldown routine, including your full-body stretches. If you're walking from your site, make an easy, meditative walk part of your cooldown after this playful session.

Workout 8: Multisite— Anywhere, USA

WORKOUT SNAPSHOT

Total time: 50 to 60 minutes.
Props: Hills and inclines, log or bench, tree limb or bar, rock or root (for balance).
Location: Just about anywhere.
Purpose: Cardio and total core, functional training.

You'll return again and again to this anytime, anywhere workout, which you can do in any park setting, in most rural settings, or on a mountain trail. You're at the point now where you can scout terrain in an instant and create a workout no matter where you are—in urban and rural environments, in the mountains, or at the beach.

Full of hill work, as well as lots of squatting, bending, lunging, twisting, pushing, and pulling, this functional workout is designed to make you physically and mentally strong as you move the way your body was intended to move—freely, with confidence and power, and in many directions!

Stage 1: Warm-Up (5 to 10 minutes)

It's still a good idea to spend time warming up before your traveling and multisite workouts, even though they are aerobically based. You want your muscles warmed up and your oxygen flowing freely. You also want to be opened up to your environment, mentally and emotionally as well as physically. Use your warm-up time to clear your mind and to engage your senses. You'll find that things flow better in your workout when you do.

Start with your basic warm-up sequence (see chapter 4), paying attention to your posture and alignment:

1. Joint lubrication
2. Reverse breath
3. High knees
4. Cardio warm-up to station 1 (5 minutes; RPE 4–5).

Get going with a fast walk or a slow jog as you head to your first station. As you move, focus on your technique: your heel-toe roll and high toes, setting the tempo of your feet by pumping your arms, and breathing properly.

Stage 2: Strengthening and Traveling

Station 1— Flat Ground

You've loosened up with a little cardio, and now it's time to do a few more warm-up exercises to "wire up" your muscles, joints, and brain for the movements and movement patterns to come in this rigorous traveling workout.

Wide-Legged Squat (1 minute)

See chapter 5.

Sumo Squat (1 minute)

See chapter 6. Control this movement through your core. Work with a range of flexibility that works for you.

Cardio Travel to Station 2 (3 minutes; RPE 5–6)

Build to an RPE of 5 to 6, a moderate effort. Engage your senses and tune in to your environment. Is the air cool on your skin? Are the leaves turning bright colors? Can you smell wood smoke or wet grass? As you near time, look for a slope with a flat spot for your upcoming squats.

Station 2— Hillside or Incline

Hill Squat (1 minute)

See chapter 6.

"Half-Tuck" Squat (30 to 60 seconds per leg)

See chapter 6. Move to the base of the hill for this exercise. Your resting leg should remain nearly straight. Remember, it has no function in this exercise. You are just getting it out of the way. Ninety-five percent of your body weight is on your downhill, support leg. Keep your hips back and do not let your bending knee drop beyond your toes.

Cardio Travel to Station 3 (2 to 3 minutes; RPE 7–8)

Read your terrain as you build your RPE to a 7 to 8, deep in your aerobic zone. You're likely hitting some tricky terrain with ups and downs and twists and turns, so make sure you keep your head up and your eyes focused at least 10 to 15 feet ahead. Take a moment to observe how much more smoothly you travel this way. As you get close to time, scout out a log, boulder, or bench for push-ups and dips.

Breathing on the Hills

When you're climbing a hill, get into a rhythmic breathing pattern in which you slowly inhale and fully exhale: easy in, easy out. You'll find, as with your reverse breath technique, that you are able to really expand your lungs and take in more air. The key here is that deep in the lower lobes of your lungs there is greater density of alveoli, the little grapelike clusters where oxygen exchange occurs, feeding your body and brain. Practice the phrase "low and slow," and your body will naturally follow along. More than anything, this technique will help you to relax and breathe properly, circulating oxygen throughout your brain and body. Your legs will burn less, and you will find you have energy to burn!

Station 3— Bench or Low Wall

"Push It–Pull It"
(1 minute)
See chapter 6.

MODIFICATION

Harder: Go inverted! Put your feet on the log, your hands on the flat ground. Pause for 1 to 3 counts at the bottom of the move before pushing back up.

Full-Body Triceps Dip
(30 to 60 seconds per leg)
See chapter 6.

MODIFICATIONS

Easier: March in place by lifting one knee up as you dip down, and then the other knee up as you dip down.

Harder: Move in slow motion. Dip down slowly, hold for a count, and slowly exhale up.

TIP: Keep your shoulders square and down, away from your ears.

Cardio Travel to Station 4
(2 to 3 minutes; RPE 7–8)

You're really feeling it now! Use this cardio block for a visualization. Feel your greatness—your strength, confidence, grace, and finesse. Now visualize that greatness: Imagine what you look like, strong and sleek, and flowing with your terrain. Step right into that vision. Become that vision. Observe how your posture improves, how you feel more focused, powerful, and graceful. That is the power of mental imagery working for you! Walk it out for 20 to 30 seconds before setting up for your next exercise.

Station 4—
Flat Ground or
Slight Incline

Forward Lunge—Walking
(1 to 2 minutes)

Begin with your standing forward lunge (see chapter 5), then walk forward, inhaling down and exhaling up. If there is an incline, travel up the hill. Walk it out for 20 to 30 seconds before moving on to your next exercise.

Full-Body Lunge
(1 to 2 minutes)
See chapter 6.

MODIFICATIONS
Easier: Perform these lunges with a long step. Lower your hips only about 1 to 2 inches and hold your arms out laterally, at shoulder height.
Harder: Bend your forward knee to 90 degrees.

Cardio Travel to Station 5
(2 to 3 minutes; RPE 7–7.5)

Shake out your body. Slowly build your RPE to 7 or 7.5. Maintain a strong posture, with your chest open, chin up, and eyes forward. Use a nice, even arm swing to maintain your tempo. Even breathing is critical to wash your body with oxygen and clear out lactic acid that has built up in your system.

About 30 seconds from time, take your RPE down to a 5 or 6.

Station 5—
Flat Ground

Standing "C" Crunch
(30 to 60 seconds per side)

See chapter 6. Lift your knee out and away from your body and then up to your chest, so that you form the letter C. For support and stability, contract your glutes in the support leg. Repeat on the other side.

Standing Cross-Over Crunch
(30 to 60 seconds per side)

This exercise targets your abdominal wall, obliques, hips, and shoulders (see chapter 6). Recover by walking it out for 30 seconds to catch your breath and clear your mind. Draw in a few deep breaths and exhale completely.

Cardio Travel to Station 6
(2 to 3 minutes; RPE 6–7)

Use this time to clear your body and mind of any tension. Take your RPE to a 6 or 7. Maintain even breathing and continue to wash your system with oxygen as you clear out any lactic acid. Stay light on your feet, maintaining an overall feeling of lightness as you move over the terrain. Imagine yourself as a light-footed animal. Think: "Bunny feet, not elephant feet." Try it—it works!

Station 6—
Rock, Root, or Bump
in the Terrain

Rock-n-Balance
(1 minute per leg)

See chapter 6.

MODIFICATIONS

Easier: Pick your foot off the ground, hold for a count of 1- and return. Continue for 30 to 60 seconds.

Harder:

• Try using a more difficult prop.
• Try it with your eyes closed.

Root Raise
(1 minute)

See chapter 6.

Cross-Training Sundays

Cross training, the rotation of sport and fitness activities on different days, is the key to preventing overuse injuries—such as tendonitis—and keeping our training effective. By rotating athletic activities, we distribute the stress of exercise to different joints and muscle groups rather than continually loading stress on one area.

Cross training also helps us avoid hitting a plateau in our training—this is when we go into "cruise control," where we are mentally and physically flat. To keep training challenging, choose an activity that you don't typically do during the week for a Sunday cross-training session. Try something completely new, such as inline skating, hiking, mountain biking, tennis, rock climbing, kayaking, or golfing. Anything that you find enjoyable and that stimulates your muscles and your brain is a great cross-training exercise.

Stage 3:
Cardio Cooldown—
Relaxed Environmental
Integration
(5 to 10 minutes)

Find a sprig of foliage, like a cluster of pine needles, a eucalyptus leaf, a bay leaf, or a fragrant flower. Curl the needles or leaf in your fingers to release the aromas. Close your eyes, breathe deeply, and connect to the core of your core. Once you feel connected, centered, and clear, begin to walk back to your starting place. Feel through your feet, breathing deeply, noticing colors, textures, and sounds. Keep the leaf in your hand so you can breathe in this aroma along the way. When you near your starting spot, walk it out until your heart rate comes all the way down. Find a quiet place to stretch and enjoy the aromas, the sights, and the sounds around you. Now that is the original aromatherapy!

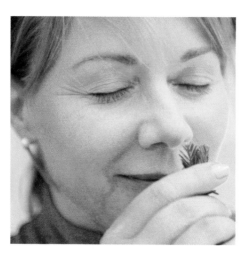

Workout 9:
Traveling—SAQ

WORKOUT SNAPSHOT

Total time: 30 to 60 minutes.

Props: No props—just terrain selection—grass, dirt, tartan track, sand, etc.

Location: Beach, track, athletic field, fire road, hillside.

Purpose: Cardio-aerobic and anaerobic conditioning; interval training with multidirectional drills for speed, agility, and quickness (SAQ).

This is a traveling workout that can take you to any number of destinations. Want to work out at the beach today? Get going. On a hillside plateau with beautiful views? No problem. With this workout, you'll warm up and get some aerobic conditioning done on your way to your destination. Once you arrive at your location, you'll do some intense interval training. You'll finish with a gentle "active recovery" by walking or lightly jogging back to your starting point.

Stage 1:
Warm-Up
(5 to 10 minutes)

A thorough warm-up is critical for this workout. Start with your regular, tried and true warm-up exercises:

TIP: Introduce your body to the work ahead. After the initial warm-up and stretching, put your body through some range-of-motion exercises for large muscle groups, such as slowly executed squats or push-ups. This helps prepare your mind, muscles, and joints for the more intense work to follow. It's also a chance for you to focus on integrating your body, mind, and environment.

1. Joint lubrication (see chapter 4)
2. Reverse breath (see chapter 4)
3. Wide-legged squats with palm-to-palm press (see chapter 5)
4. Push-ups (see chapter 5)
5. High knees (see chapter 4)
6. Lateral Leg Press—Shuffle

To turn your lateral leg press (see chapter 5) into a "shuffle"—take off slowly to the right, pressing firmly through the arch of your left foot. Maintain a strong upper body, and do not collapse at the waist.

Stage 2: Interval Training

Before beginning your interval work, mark out a stretch of grass, dirt, or sand about 30 to 50 yards long. As you warm up, scout the terrain for any divots, bumps, holes, sprinklers, or broken glass. Make sure you know what is underfoot so you can feel confident moving quickly across the terrain during your drills.

Warm-Up Drills (4 to 5 minutes)

Alternate a 1-minute drill with 1 minute of active recovery.

FAQ on SAQ

Why Speed, Agility, and Quickness (SAQ)?
Remember how quick and agile you were as a child? You ran flat out on the playground, darting and dodging the other kids in games of tag. You were having fun, but you were also building valuable sports and fitness skills.

SAQ is fundamental to athletic performance and comprises the hallmarks of every top-notch athlete. It's true, some people are born with a natural ability to move swiftly and weave with precision and grace. Everyone, though, has the potential to increase their power and sharpen their response time through training. That's because the body learns by doing—including your body!

What Is SAQ?

SAQ workouts consist of short, intense drills that require you to accelerate or decelerate quickly while moving backward, forward, or side to side. SAQ improves balance, power, and neuromuscular firing patterns so that your movements become fast, dynamic, and precise. You'll notice improvements in your response time and your ability to change direction lightning fast—as in basketball, tennis, skiing, and soccer.

Do I Need SAQ?

If you like to participate in sports like golf, tennis, skiing, or even table tennis, you'll want to listen up. These and many other sports are explosive—and explosive sports must be trained explosively. Whether you are sprinting, rock climbing, or hitting a golf ball, there is always a critical moment where you need extra power between the waist and the knees.

This training helps protect you from injury when you are trying new sports or adding new challenges to your workouts. If you teach your muscles to fire contrary to the way they are used to, you will prepare your tendons, ligaments, muscles, and joints for the unexpected, and this will help prevent injury.

Oh, and SAQ is a whole lot of fun, too!

What Is SAQ Training?

Before you start a SAQ program, it's important to have a solid athletic base of strength, cardiovascular endurance, and flexibility.

Proper warm-up is a must. It takes a minimum of 10 minutes to properly warm up muscles, ligaments, and joints. Try light jogging and other rhythmic-type movements like step-ups and jumping jacks.

Shoe quality cannot be overemphasized. Be sure that your footwear fits well, is supportive, and is made for multidirectional movement.

Movement quality is paramount. Maintain proper execution and muscle control at all times.

Less is more. Shorten the duration of the actual workouts to 20 to 30 minutes, with full recovery between sets.

Remember: The emphasis is on going fast!

Lateral Leg Press—Shuffle (2 minutes)

Take off laterally to the right, building speed by pressing firmly through the arch of your left foot. The lower your hips, the more challenging it is.

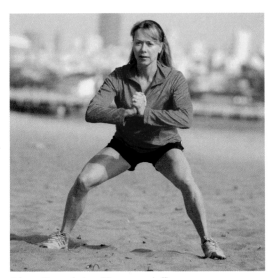

Take a wide step for lateral leg press—shuffle

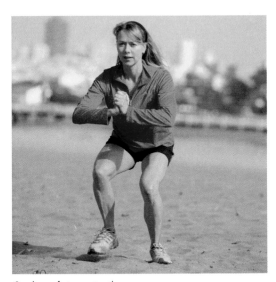

Stay low as feet come together

Maintain a strong upper body and do not collapse at the waist.

Backward-to-Forward Jog (2 minutes)

Take off, moving backward with a "toe-heel" roll—plant your toes first and roll through the entire foot. Keep your hips low and pump your arms, building up your speed. Jog forward to the start and repeat.

Interval Cycle (1 to 10 minutes)

Alternate 60 seconds of intense drill training with 30 to 60 seconds of active recovery.

Lateral Shuffle—3-Hop Stop (3 minutes)

Take off laterally, shuffle three times, stop, and hop around 180 degrees to face the other direction. Shuffle three times, now leading with the other foot, stop, and hop around to face the original direction. Repeat the entire length of the field. Jog back to the start and repeat.

Diagonal Stride (3 minutes)

With your right foot, take a long step into a diagonal stride—your left elbow forward and in line with your right knee. Press off the big-toe-to-arch of your left foot, to engage the adductors of your inner thigh. Step your feet together. Alternate with your other leg, using your

Power Words

Key words or "power words" are useful tools in helping to stay focused during clutch moments and intense phases of your workout. One or two meaningful words can provide you with a quick burst of motivation and inspiration, just when you need it most. If you feel yourself tensing up, "low and slow" can help you relax. If you need a little extra push, try "dig deep!"

arms to set the tempo and to assist you with power in your stride. Within a few strides you will begin to pick up speed, and this will become more like bounding. Recover with a light jog back. Repeat.

Shuffle Run (3 minutes)

Take off running or sprinting for about 10 yards, touch the ground, and run back to the start, touching the ground there. Take off running again for about 20 yards, touch the ground, turn around, and run back to the start. Take off running for about 30 yards, touch the ground, and return to the start. You get the picture! Continue for the length of the field. Recover and repeat.

Recovery Lap (2 to 3 minutes)

Take some time to gradually lower your heart rate with a light jog or a fast walk. Remember, you don't want to suddenly stop because your heart is beating at a high rate and all of that blood needs to be circulated. A sudden stop will cause the blood to pool in your limbs—called venous pooling. It creates pressure in your body and can also lead to broken capillaries and varicose veins!

Interval Cycle (2 to 10 minutes)

Alternate 60 seconds of intense drill training with 30 to 60 seconds of active recovery.

Speed and Quickness Drill (3 minutes)

With these drills, focus on "three-step" speed: Run flat out for about 10 yards, shuffle to the right three steps, and then shuffle to the left three steps. Repeat.

Big "T" Drill (3 minutes)

Enscribe a huge letter T in the dirt or sand. If you can't trace in the earth, use cones, rocks, sticks—or just your imag-

TIP: To get into the rhythm of this drill, think: slide, slide; back, back, back; forward, forward, forward; slide, slide.

The Secret of Interval Training

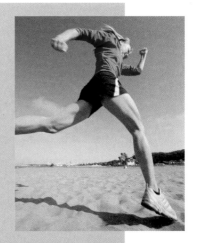

I'll let you in on a little secret that trainers and coaches have known for a long time: Adding interval training to your workout can help you boost your fat-blasting capabilities while you shorten your workout! All "interval training" means is short bursts of anaerobic, high-intensity activity followed by longer periods of moderate or low-intensity activity. One study showed that people who incorporated interval training into their routines lost *nine times* more body fat than those who chose to do only aerobic exercise.

Interval training will stoke your metabolism. You'll burn more calories and blast more fat during your workout, and also after you've put your running shoes away. The key is fuel burning. Think about driving, and imagine you are low on fuel. Do you punch the gas pedal? No, you finesse your way to the gas station with light taps on the accelerator. Why? Because you know that quick bursts will burn more gas. Our bodies are the same way. Interval training simply burns more fuel. In these workouts, you're using both your aerobic and anaerobic systems—that's the one with oxygen and the one without. You use up more oxygen, burn up more sugar, and blast through more calories.

Once you've been consistent with your program for six to eight weeks, you can start adding intervals. You can incorporate interval training a couple of times per week, if you like. This change-up to your training routine will also keep your body from going on autopilot when it gets too accustomed to your regular workout.

Interval training tips:

- Try going hard for 1 minute and easy for 2 minutes—that's interval training.
- Find hills and steps. Push your intensity up the hill and recover on the return trip down.
- Use the local track. Sprint the straights and jog or walk the turns. Instead of a timer, you can use landmarks—phone poles, city blocks, mailboxes, and street signs.

ination—to create a T as big as you'd like. Shuffle laterally across the top of the T to the middle. Run backward along the leg of the T. Run forward up the leg, then shuffle laterally left. Side shuffle back to the start, across the top of the T. Repeat two to five times.

Four-Corner Drill (3 minutes)

Take four rocks and make a square, placing the rocks about 10 yards apart. Place a stick, pinecone, or rock in the middle. Run from the corner to the stick on the inside, run back to the same corner, then run up to the next corner. Repeat. Move as quickly as you can, trying to get faster with each drill.

Stage 3: Recovery, Cooldown, and Flexibility

Shake your legs out, breathe deeply, and start walking slowly to circulate oxy-gen into your system and to relieve any burning or fatigue you feel in your legs. As the burning subsides, steadily build your RPE to 7 or 7.5 for the trip back.

At your starting point, find a spot to stretch. You may want to begin the stretching phase of your cooldown with a leg drain (prop your feet up on a wall or tree) before starting your full-body stretches.

Full-body stretches (see chapter 4):
- Hip flexors
- Hamstrings
- Quadriceps
- Inner thighs (adductors)
- Calves
- Chest, shoulders, and biceps
- Upper back and rear shoulders
- Torso

CHAPTER 8

Quickies

Short on time? These workouts pack a lot of activity into very little time—providing strength, flexibility, and cardiovascular benefits in just a few minutes. These are the workouts you turn to when you think, "I'm way too busy today to exercise." You can slip any of these seven workouts into a spare 10 minutes. Trust me, putting in that 10 minutes really does make a difference. It's a whole lot better for your mind and body than doing nothing at all.

By this point, you will more than likely be familiar with most of the following exercises. If you want a workout that is slightly longer than 10 minutes— say, 20 minutes—then run through the selected workout twice or do two of the quickies. You can also use this list as a kind of cheat sheet, so that when you are short on time, you can still fit in a mini workout. Doing one or two of these

exercises is time well spent: Split squat, push it–pull it, full-body triceps dip, TVA/ab flattener—you can knock that combination out in mere minutes!

Choose from these seven workouts based on your mood, your location, and the type of quick challenge you'd like to take on:

1. Full-body bench workout
2. Total body tree workout
3. "One-spot" lower body
4. Full-body express
5. Restorative workout
6. Proprioception and balance
7. High-intensity fat-blaster workout

All seven workouts combine super efficiency, convenience, and fun, with the Outdoor Fitness BodyMind challenges you're used to getting in your longer sessions.

Warm-Up

Always begin each workout with the Outdoor Fitness warm-up routine (5 minutes), as discussed in chapter 4:

1. Joint lubrication
2. Reverse breath
3. Posture check
4. High knees
5. Cardio warm-up (3 to 5 minutes), including a fast walk to the location and step-ups once you're there.

Time for all warm-ups has been included for these routines, with the exception that some need additional warm-up exercises that mimic the movements in the upcoming workouts.

Quickie 1: Full-Body Bench Workout (10 minutes)

The only thing you need to complete this workout is a bench, block, or sturdy stump. That's it! This total-body session targets all of your major muscle groups. It will also get your heart pumping. You'll walk away from this workout fully oxygenated, with a rosy glow.

Perform each exercise for 60 to 90 seconds:

1. Step-up
2. Lateral step-up
3. Wide-legged squat
4. Full-body press
5. Full-body triceps dip
6. TVA/ab flattener

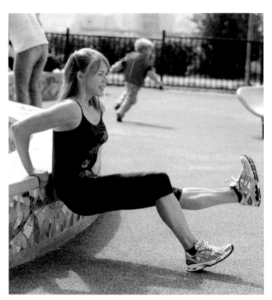

Full-body triceps dip

Quickie 2: Total-Body Tree Workout (10 minutes)

If you can sneak out for 10 minutes to a local park—or your backyard—this total-body workout will reward you with a great muscle-strengthening session.

Perform each exercise for 60 to 90 seconds per side:

1. Tree sit
2. Tree stand—upper body
3. Tree stand—lower body
4. One-armed press
5. "Reverse" pull-up

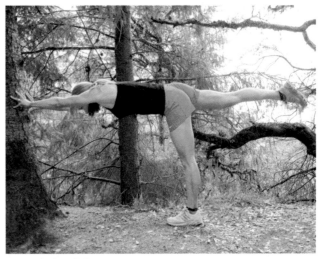

Tree stand—lower body

Quickie 3: "One-Spot" Lower Body (10 minutes)

Short on time *and* space? No problem. You can complete this well-rounded lower-body workout on your front porch in 10 minutes or less.

Perform 15 to 25 repetitions of each of the following exercises:

Warm-up Exercises

1. High knees
2. Step-up

Exercises

1. Split squat
2. Reverse lunge
3. Standing forward lunge
4. "Half-tuck" squat
5. Sumo squat

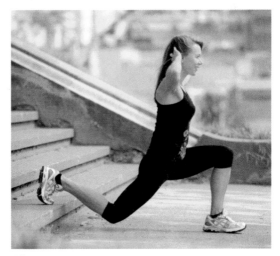

Split squat

Quickie 4:
Full-Body Express
(10 minutes)

This session works everywhere for everyone. Whether you're a beginner or an experienced athlete, whether you live in the heart of the city or the outskirts of town, you can help firm up your body in 10 minutes with this super-efficient session. This workout sculpts arms, tightens abs, and tones legs—and you never have to go near a gym!

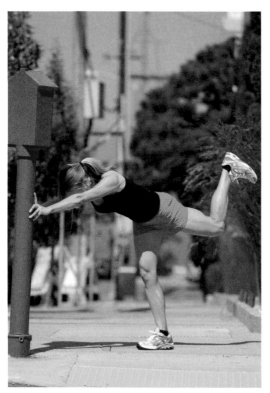

Tree stand with heel press

Do 2 sets of 10 to 20 reps of each move, unless otherwise noted. Warm up with 5 minutes of walking or jogging, and be sure to stretch afterward.

1. Split squat
2. "Palm-to-palm" pull-up
3. "Tree stand" with heel press
4. Triceps dip
5. Standing "C" crunch

Afterward, do a full-body stretch.

Quickie 5:
Restorative Workout
(15 to 20 minutes)

Maybe you're feeling a little fatigued or sore, but you still want to do some sort of refreshing exercise. Imagine completing a relaxing series of flowing, slow-motion movements in an aromatic grove as you watch the first rays of the morning sun and listen to the sounds of waves lapping against the beach. This gentle, single-site workout can be done at a beach or a park, by a riverside or a plaza fountain, or in a grassy field. Its stimulating and soothing exercises will clear your mind, relax you, and get your blood pumping.

Remember, this workout is about relaxation and awareness, so find an open space in a quiet, pleasant area.

Breathe, feel your body, and integrate yourself with the environment around you—setting yourself up for a perfect day.

Warm-up (5 minutes)

1. Joint lubrication
2. Reverse breath
3. Posture check
4. High knees

Exercises

Spend 60 to 90 seconds at each station and perform each exercise in "slow motion" by adding a second or 2 to each phase of the movement.

1. Full-body press
2. Wide-legged squat
3. Reverse lunge
4. Lateral leg press
5. Single-leg dip
6. TVA/ab flattener
7. Aqua

Repeat all seven exercises once more with internal cues, including *eyes closed.*

Cooldown

1. Full-body clench and release
2. Flexibility

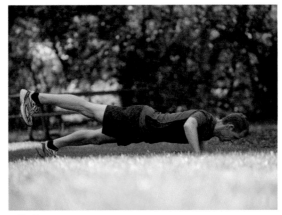

Full-body press

Quickie 6: Proprioception and Balance (10 minutes)

You can do this balance session just about anywhere. You can also easily integrate this short session into any other workout. Look around your backyard or neighborhood park for the following props for your balance routine:

• Rock or small bump in the ground
• Curb or root
• Tree or wall

Most of these balance exercises also strengthen the lower body. There is some correlation between balance exercises and strength-training exercises, so it's a "two for one": You get strength and toning with the added benefit of balance training.

Perform 2 sets of each exercise for 60 to 90 seconds:

1. Proprioception exercise: see chapter 1.
2. Rock-n-balance
3. Single-leg dip
4. Calf raise
5. Tree stand—upper body (with or without the tree)

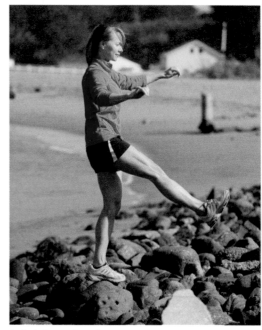

Rock-n-balance—foot in front

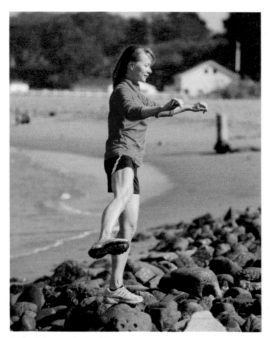

Rock-n-balance—foot to side

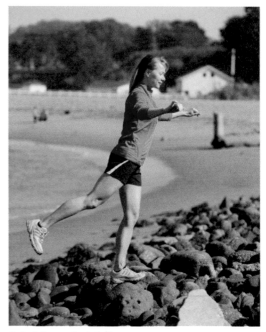

Rock-n-balance—foot behind

Quickie 7: High-Intensity Fat-Blaster Workout (20 minutes)

Maybe you've hit a plateau in your weight-loss program or you're trying to slim down fast for a special occasion — or maybe you ate a little more than you planned to last night. Maybe you'd just like to blow off a little steam. This is the workout for you! This session uses intervals (repeated short, intense bursts of effort) to maximize the amount of calories you burn. This challenging session can be done as a single-site, multisite, or traveling workout. The workout calls for hills, but you can also incorporate stairs or bleachers, or a track, in place of a road or path over hilly terrain.

Competitive athletes have relied on interval training and conditioning for a long time because of the results it delivers. You'll find interval work an effective, efficient, and fun way to mix up your training sessions and burn a heck of a lot of calories — during and *after* the workout!

Your intervals will involve short periods of high-intensity effort immediately followed by active recovery. Be sure to complete a thorough warm-up before you start your intervals.

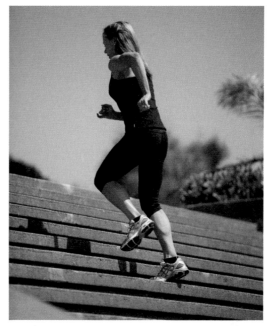
Intervals using steps

Warm-up (8 minutes)

1. Joint lubrication and breathing exercise (1 minute)
2. High knees (1 minute)
3. Walk to jog, slowly building to RPE 6–7 (5 minutes)
4. Sumo squat (1 minute)

Intervals

1. Crescendos RPE 1–8
   Just like in music!
• Start up the hill building your intensity, mentally and physically clicking off your RPE scale, from 1, 2, 3, 4 . . . to 8.

• When you get to the top, don't stop! Turn right around and make slalom turns as if you are skiing across the fall line on the return trip down the hill. This will take the impact out of your knees and you'll work on agility.

2. Lateral Leg Press
12–20 reps per side

It's time to take it sideways!

• Start low and stay low, pressing through the arch of your bottom foot and *pushing*. If it gets too tough, run up the rest of the way.
• When you get to the top, *don't* turn around. Take it backwards down the hill. If it's too slick or gravelly don't go backwards—instead use slalom turns to get yourself to the base.

3. Crescendos RPE 8.5–9

Repeat this interval up the hill, this time building to a greater RPE level of 8.5–9. Make slalom turns on the return trip down.

4. Diagonal Stride
20–50 reps RPE 8–9

• When you do these, think skater—get low and use your glutes and legs powerfully. Use powerful arms to set a fast tempo.
• Face up the hill. With your left foot, take a long step up the hill, into a diagonal stride—put your right elbow forward and in line with your left knee.
• Lean into the hill, with your body weight evenly distributed between both feet. Lower your hips until you can feel pressure under the heel and arch of your left foot and the big toe and ball of your right foot.
• Exhale as you press off the big toe-to-arch of the right foot to engage the adductors of the inner thigh.
• Step your feet together, and alternate with the other leg.

5. Hill Sprint RPE 8.5–9

• It's time to just let 'er rip!
• Start fast and keep going, reaching an RPE of 8.5–9.
• On your return trip, use fatigue to your advantage: take it backwards down the hill, so you have to practice touch and focus.

Repeat—If you've got the time!

Otherwise, walk it out. Be sure to stretch your legs as part of your cooldown.

TIP: To increase your speed, use your arms for power, push through your glutes, and fire firmly off the back toes.

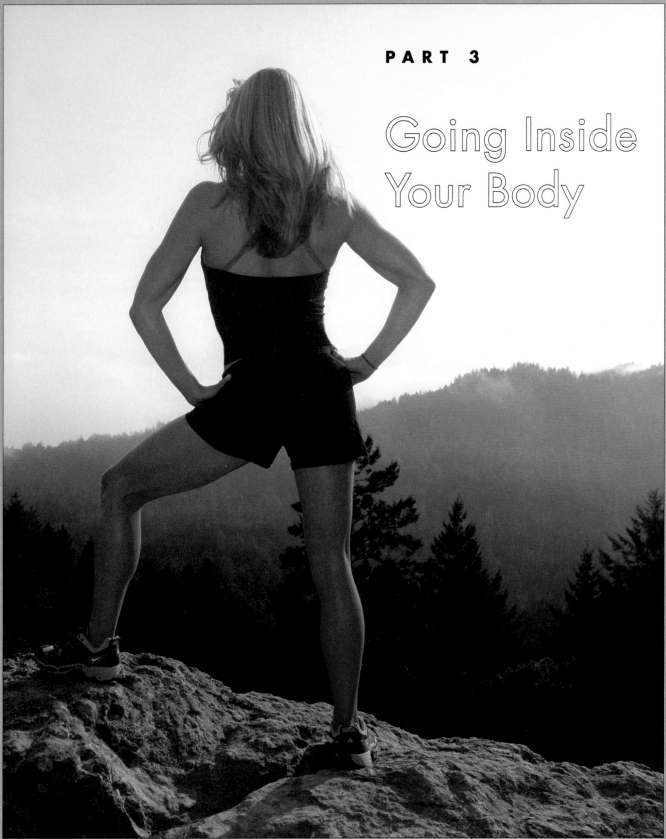

PART 3

Going Inside
Your Body

MITCHEL SHENKER

CHAPTER 9

Taking Care of Your Body by Eating the Outdoor Fitness Way

Good nutrition is an integral element of Outdoor Fitness. My approach to eating is balanced, makes the most of high-nutrient foods, doesn't take too much planning, and will keep you satisfied and support your workouts. It's a way to eat with pleasure and variety through the seasons and the years, for a lifetime of health and well-being.

So many of us begin a fitness program because we want to lose weight. You're about to learn that changing your body composition—losing fat and gaining muscle—is the true key to getting and staying trim, fit, and healthy. As a personal trainer, I know that concern and confusion about diet are common for people, especially in the beginning of their program. People start out frustrated and usually feel anxious and desperate to make changes. "I can't fit into

my clothes." "I am fat!" "I want to look good for my wedding." "I have my high school reunion coming up."

Beneath all these reasons is the same deeper motivation. We all want to *feel* good. These events simply act as the catalyst for change. People like you who start Outdoor Fitness make a wonderful discovery: You can feel good and feel motivated, be lean, strong, healthy, and vibrant all the time. You don't have to crash diet for a special occasion or feel nervous when you pull out your favorite pair of shorts at the beginning of the summer. Changing your body composition and maintaining your healthy body—and yes, losing weight—are entirely possible without feeling miserable and deprived. You just need the right information.

As part of the Outdoor Fitness program, you'll learn to eat for better body composition. When you achieve—and maintain—a positive ratio between muscle and fat, your body will be strong and lean. You'll have the energy to perform and the ability to think and focus clearly. You'll even out your blood sugar, and you'll feel good all day—without the mood swings or the late-afternoon energy crash. You'll look and feel healthy, fit, and vibrant. Well-being will flow out of your pores. If your goal is to gain muscle and lose fat, or if you are on a maintenance program, my nutrition guidelines will deliver results.

These guidelines are based on the Outdoor Fitness research study I developed. The study was monitored by Dr. Adrian Rawlinson of California Pacific Orthopedics and Sports Medicine Group in San Francisco. Participants in our 60-day body composition makeover saw striking results:

- Losses of 7 to 15 pounds of pure body fat
- Fat loss of 3 to 7 percent
- Increased muscle and tone
- Decrease in daily stress
- Increased feelings of happiness and well-being

In this chapter you will learn about body composition, the elements of nutrition, and the components of a balanced, moderate, nutrient-rich diet. You'll bring all this new knowledge together in an 11-point game plan that's easy to follow

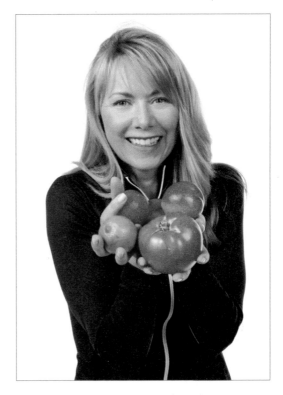

and suitable for both weight loss and maintenance.

Body Composition

Understanding your body composition is an important first step in remaking your health and well-being. What is body composition? Simply, it's a measurement of your body's individual ratio of body fat to lean body mass. Body fat is found under the skin, laced between your muscles, and it acts as a cushion between your organs. Lean body mass consists of everything but fat: muscles, bones, organs, and blood.

Health problems occur when there is too much body fat, and also when there is too little body fat. Too much body fat, especially when located around the abdomen, increases the risk of many diseases, including type 2 diabetes, high blood pressure, stroke, heart disease, and certain cancers. Too little body fat is linked to problems with normal healthy functioning in both men and women, and it can lead to problems with reproduction in women. Whether you're a competitive athlete or an exercise enthusiast, your performance as well as your health can be improved with optimal body composition—not too much body fat, but not too little.

Ditch the Scale

Here's some good news: You can stop glaring at your bathroom scale. Knowing your body composition ratio is a much more accurate and objective measure of health and fitness than your weight.

Weight is an unreliable and often deceptive indicator in measuring your baseline health and the effectiveness of your fitness program because your body weight can change by a lot—day to day, hour by hour—simply from the foods you eat. A salty meal can leave you bloated and unable to button your favorite jeans, and a night of unhealthy foods can leave you constipated and heavier.

When you're working out to improve your health and fitness, as well as shrink your waistline, you need a reliable way to measure your progress. Again, body composition wins out over body weight. As you lose fat, you'll be gaining muscle—in fact, it is not uncommon to gain weight when you start strength training before you eventually begin to lose weight.

Does Muscle Weigh More than Fat?

No! A pound of muscle is equal to a pound of fat. The difference between muscle and fat is in volume: Body fat takes up about three to four times the volume of muscle. This is why you'll tighten and shrink your body as you get fit, even if your weight isn't dropping dramatically.

The Limits of BMI

You're probably familiar with the body mass index, or BMI. A common yardstick for weight and health, BMI is a measurement system based on body weight and height that is used frequently by doctors, nutritionists, and other health professionals. Both body composition and BMI seek to measure the same thing, for the same reason: the amount of fat in your body as an assessment of your health. Body composition, however, provides a much more accurate measurement of body fat than BMI. The reason? Measuring weight against height doesn't take into account where your body weight comes from. You might have a lot of muscle and a very healthy amount of fat but be considered "overweight" by the height/weight charts used to measure BMI. Of course, the opposite can also be true. Your body can carry a lot of fat and little muscle. In this case, you might not register as overweight on the BMI, but your body is "overfat" nonetheless.

Measuring Your Body Composition

With a few simple measurements, you can assess your body composition on your own. All you need is a tape measure. You'll use the measurements to calculate the waist-to-hip ratio (WHR), which is a useful tool for determining your fat distribution and gauging health. Once you've figured this, you can refer to it as you track your progress during the phases of Outdoor Fitness. Be prepared to see some numbers drop!

Waist-to-Hip Ratio (WHR)

- Take your waist measurement. The tape should go around the narrowest part of your waist. Relax, exhale, and take the measurement.
- Take your hip measurement around the widest part of your buttocks. Make sure the tape is snug against your skin, but not tight.
- Divide your waist measurement by your hip measurement to arrive at your WHR.

For example, if your waist is 28 inches and your hips are 36 inches, your WHR is 0.78.

What Does My WHR Mean?

Generally, a healthy WHR is below 0.9 for men and below 0.8 for women—anything over 1.0 means your waistline is wider than your hips. Waist sizes over 40 inches for men or over 35 inches for women are associated with greater health risk.

5 Steps to Better Body Composition

1. Use the power of your mind and think about your body composition. What do you want it to be? Visualize that healthy, fit, well-proportioned self.

2. Write down and revisit your goals often. Be sure to focus on *why* you'd like to achieve them. Be specific.

3. Plan ahead. During the first few weeks, plan all your meals, including snacks. Write out your food plan first thing in the morning and follow that plan throughout the day.

4. Organize your exercise, including rest days. Put it down on your calendar, just as you would an appointment. Include two to three days of strength training, three to four days of cardiovascular conditioning, a day of cross training, and a day of rest.

5. Measure your body composition. Retest yourself after 8 to 12 weeks and record your progress.

The Belly Fat Problem

High levels of cortisol—the stress hormone—have been shown to contribute to higher levels of fat in the body, especially deep belly fat. Many factors can lift your levels of cortisol—too much stress, a lack of sleep, smoking, and drinking alcohol. Science has shown that abdominal fat, especially the deep layer, called visceral fat, is the most troublesome kind of fat. It is associated with diabetes and heart disease. This visceral fat behaves differently than other fats because it's more metabolically active.

Here's the good news: Because this deep belly fat is so metabolically active, it's easier to budge. Here's an easy test you can do to find out if it's time to whittle your middle.

Measure your waist. Men with a waist over 40 inches and women with a waist of more than 35 inches should work on ridding themselves of belly fat. What's the best way to get rid of visceral fat? If you said sit-ups, think again. Crunches and core exercises are great for toning and strengthening, but they don't burn fat like cardio. To trim your middle, focus on your cardio workouts. Get your heart pumping in your aerobic zone for at least 20 minutes to start, and work up to 60 or more minutes. Practice mental clearing and meditation exercises during your cardio—great tools to help you reduce your stress levels.

Eating to Improve Your Body Composition

Losing fat and maintaining your ideal body composition is not about deprivation; it is about creating healthy habits that you can maintain and incorporate into your lifestyle. With these four principles—eating well, eating often, using portion control, and eating the right combination of foods—you have a road map for a lifetime of healthy eating and weight control. You'll start out by losing fat and gaining muscle. Once you've reached your body composition goal, you can use these same strategies to maintain your body composition and weight, as well as preserve and protect your health. The meal templates and food lists in the Food Facts section offer you structure and many fantastic, healthy foods to choose from in creating your new diet.

Eat Well

Simple, whole foods are your ticket to a great body, inside and out. Fruits, vegetables, and whole grains can be found in abundance wherever you live, and these foods should be the foundation of your everyday eating. By basing your diet on these foods, you'll create nutrient-dense meals without loading up on calories. Here are a few steps that can help you make the most of simple, whole-food eating without getting bored:

Eat a variety of foods. Choose vegetables and fruits of many colors. A colorful diet is also a well-balanced diet. Take a look in your fridge. Do you see an assortment of red, yellow, green, white, purple, and orange? Your eyes can help you manage your diet by keeping a variety of whole foods on hand.

Eat seasonally and locally. Fresh tomatoes in winter? Not if you live in New England. Buying locally grown foods and eating foods in season help keep variety in your diet and allow you to enjoy food at its freshest, when it's packed with the most nutrients.

Pile on the vegetables. Be sure to add an extra serving of vegetables to at least two of your daily meals. You'll fill up on the fresh stuff before you have a chance to crave anything that's fried or processed.

Drink your water. You need at least 8 to 10 glasses of water per day. Avoid sodas, energy drinks, and other sugary beverages. Keep alcohol to a minimum—one drink per day for women and two drinks per day for men is considered moderate. In combination with fresh natural foods, plenty of water will leave you feeling satiated and energized.

Riding the Roller Coaster

I learned the hard way how processed foods and sugar affect mood and blood sugar levels and cause fat gain. I was one of those people who got caught up in the low-fat craze. I became obsessed with reading food labels and sleuthing my way through the market in search of "zero fat." From breads, cookies, and crackers to puddings, yogurts, and sodas, I found plenty of what I was looking for: no-fat foods full of sugar and stripped of any nutritional value.

At this time in my life, I was an athlete, skier, mountain biker, and inline skater. I made my living as an action sports model shooting for magazines like *Men's Journal, Mountain Bike,* and *Skiing,* and companies like Salomon, Rollerblade, and Scott, and also modeling sportswear for Patagonia, Ralph Lauren, and Fila. I had to be in shape and look like a fit athlete. The way I was eating caused a couple of big problems. My no-fat diet left me tired and fatigued. After eating, I'd feel moody, tired, irritated, and sometimes dizzy, and I'd often take a nap after lunch. I also got fat. I craved crackers and bread and anything sweet. Soon I found myself on a roller coaster that went like this: I'd be hired for a modeling job that required small outfits, and I would diet like a madwoman, eating only crackers, toast, nonfat yogurt, some vegetables, and water with lemon in it. My roommates would run for cover during this time. I never understood why until a couple of years later after we'd all moved our separate ways. "You were a bear, Tina," one of them said. "You were snappish and unhappy."

Yikes! It wasn't until I read a popular diet book and met with a nutritionist that I learned what was happening to me—I had a classic case of insulin resistance. With recommendations from my nutritionist and my own research, I made some big changes to my diet. I cut out all the processed stuff, and after one meal I started to feel better, less fatigued and sleepy. I knew then I had a problem eating processed foods.

In the years since, I've learned a new way to eat. I've learned that food is meant to energize, heal, and build my body, and most of all, I learned that I should *enjoy* eating! My diet is one based on fresh, mostly seasonal and organic food. I now crave color—red tomatoes, yellow peppers, deep green lettuces, and whatever I can find at the farmer's market or in the local produce aisle. There is also an excitement about eating food so fresh—it has life inside! Scientists are still learning about the healing properties of phytonutrients found in the colorful produce we eat.

Keep It Clean

Part of eating well means keeping away from the pesticides, herbicides, and fungicides that contaminate so much of our food supply. To improve the cleanliness of your food, try to do the following:

- Buy organic food whenever possible.
- Be selective. Avoid produce that is bruised or punctured or that has mold spots.
- Wash your produce in water. Use a scrub brush to clean the exterior and rinse thoroughly.
- Scrub the outside of melons with water or a produce wash and rinse thoroughly before cutting the rinds. The blade of your knife can transfer contaminants to the flesh of the fruit.
- For waxed produce like cucumbers, rinse in cool water before peeling.

Practice Portion Control

In Outdoor Fitness, we don't count calories. Portion control takes the place of calorie counting, a simple method that you can use anytime, anywhere—no scribbling, no calculators, no numbers to remember. This doesn't mean we ignore calories—you've got to understand the caloric value of the food you eat—but practicing portion control is the easiest and most effective way to keep your plate in balance.

Portion sizes have spun out of control: Everything is supersized. I believe this out-of-control portioning is part of the reason why more than 65 percent of Americans are overweight. We've simply forgotten what reasonable portions look like, and most of us are unaware of exactly how much we're eating. A great way to help cut back on calories, however, is to use a smaller plate. A study published in the *American Journal of Preventive Medicine* has demonstrated that reducing the size of your plate, bowl, cup, or spoon can actually help you control what you eat and diminish your portions. Participants in the study— all nutrition experts themselves—served themselves 31 percent more food when using the larger plate of two offered to them. People who used the larger bowl and spoon ate nearly 57 percent more than those who opted for the smaller bowl and utensil.

Some portion sizes to use as guidelines follow. Create a plate based on these, and you'll never find yourself mindlessly overeating:

- A serving of protein is about the size of the palm of your hand. Just the palm—not your fingers, too!
- A serving of carbohydrate is about the size of your fist. Think of a small apple.
- For chopped fruits, vegetables, and cooked whole grains, a serving is about what you can hold in your cupped hand, roughly ½ cup.
- For whole-grain cereal, and berries, a serving is about the size of a baseball, 1 cup.
- A serving of fats and oils is a small amount; use these foods sparingly. One tablespoon of oil is 14 grams of fat and approximately 100 calories.
- A serving of peanut butter, 2 tablespoons, is about the size of a walnut in its shell.
- For hard fats, like butter and cheese, a serving is a pat of butter or the tip of your index finger.

Eat Frequently

Eating early and often creates a metabolic reaction in your body. By eating small, well-portioned meals throughout the day, you continually stoke and strengthen your body's engine.

Good eating habits begin with breakfast. Think about what happens when you skip breakfast: You might not feel hungry until noon or even later, but once you start eating—watch out. You're likely to overeat for the rest of the day.

On the other hand, if you start your day with breakfast and continue to eat frequently throughout the day, you never give your body the experience of feeling ravenous. You gently rev your metabolism all day long as you feed your body good food in reasonable portions. Eat every few hours, and you will maintain and gain lean muscle mass and burn excess fat. You'll stop cravings and sharp hunger, and you'll have more energy. You'll even think more clearly and be less grouchy!

To keep your metabolism going all day long, try the following:

- Eat breakfast within two hours of waking up.
- Eat five to six times throughout the day. This should include three meals and two or three snacks.
- Do not let more than four hours pass between one meal and the next.
- Choose a time in the evening to end all eating. The best time is two to

three hours before you plan to go to bed. Don't worry if you feel hungry; that's your body telling you it's burning calories. You'll soon grow accustomed to your new routine.

Combine Food Types

Every meal you eat should have a combination of protein, carbohydrates, and fat. You need all these elements in your daily diet in order to feel satisfied, think clearly, and to keep your energy up—not to mention the energy you'll need for your Outdoor Fitness workouts. However, in the case of protein, carbohydrates, and fats, there are good choices and not-so-good choices. The food list in the Food Facts section breaks down the good and the bad of proteins, carbs, and fats, so you'll never have to guess what's the best choice for your body. Later in this chapter, you'll learn more

Eating the Outdoor Fitness Way: A Sample Day

Breakfast
Egg-white scramble (made with three to four egg whites and one yolk, chopped veggies, and 2 tablespoons of salsa)

Midmorning Snack
½ cup low-fat cottage cheese
½ cup blueberries

Lunch
Grilled chicken salad with 1 tablespoon of vinaigrette or lemon juice

Afternoon Snack
Small handful of almonds and apple slices or a no-sugar protein shake

Dinner
Salmon
Dinner salad with 1 tablespoon of light dressing
Broccoli with lemon

about what makes up these foods, what they do for your body, and how best to combine them for body composition, fat loss, and weight maintenance.

The Straight Skinny on Fat Loss

Unfortunately, when it comes to losing fat, exercise alone is simply not enough. To lose one pound of fat, you must burn through 3,500 calories. In the Outdoor Fitness program, you're not required to count calories—instead, you'll be managing your food intake by using portion control (and how you feel). However, it is important that you understand the caloric density (content) of the foods you eat, as well as what constitutes a serving size.

For fat loss to occur, it is important that you consume a reduced number of overall calories. But you must keep eating! Consuming too few calories is harmful to your body and ultimately impedes permanent, lasting weight loss. Women should consume no fewer than 1,200 calories per day, and men should consume no fewer than 1,500 calories per day.

With practice and a little attention, you'll get very good at eating the right foods in the right amounts at the right time.

Know Your Basal Metabolic Rate (BMR)

There's no quick fix, no magic pill, and definitely no shortcuts to lasting weight loss. There is, however, one piece of good news: There's no mystery to what it takes to drop pounds and inches. The method is simple: burn more calories than you consume. In essence, it all boils down to calories in versus calories out.

To win at this numbers game, you need to know how many calories you burn just by living your normal day, which is called your basal metabolic rate (BMR). This number, which is different for everyone, represents all the energy required in a 24-hour period to beat your heart, grow your hair, and just be alive. Your BMR measures resting energy expenditure—that is, how many calories your body needs just to function on a daily basis. This number does not include activities beyond normal bodily functions like the beating of your heart, the functioning of your internal organs, and the blinking of your eyes. Obviously, exercise contributes additional calorie output, which you can factor into your food plan once you know your BMR.

Here's a simple way to make a ballpark assessment of your BMR: multiply your weight by the number 10. For example: You weigh 150 pounds. Multiply that by 10, and your BMR is 1,500—which means that it takes 1,500 calories per day for your body just to function. If you create a deficit of 500 calories per day, you'll lose a pound per week. Or, even better, exercise to burn 300 to 500 calories, and eat 200 fewer calories per day, and you'll see even faster results.

Eating Intuitively

A remarkable thing happens when you eliminate the junk from your diet: The cravings for fatty, sugar-laden, and salty snacks will disappear. Then, when you do eat them, your new body will rebel in no uncertain terms, leaving you feeling unwell. Free of the cravings for processed foods, your body will start to crave natural, healthful whole foods. Soon the gap between the foods you want and the foods you should eat will disappear. Your intuitive sense of what your body needs will help keep you on the right track, eating simply, often, and for long-term good health.

Nutrition

There's no substitute for knowledge when it comes to learning how to eat well for a lifetime. Learn the basics of food and nutrition, and you take a big step forward in taking control of your health

and reshaping your body composition. Take ownership of the choices you make by being informed. The array of food choices is vast—often dizzying—but with a rock-solid understanding of what you're choosing to put in your body, you'll see how the choices you make can add up to a balanced, energy- and health-boosting diet. In general, all food can be broken down into macronutrients and micronutrients.

Macronutrients

Macronutrients are protein, fats, and carbohydrates. They provide your body with calories for energy, metabolism, and growth. *Macro* simply means you'll consume them in large amounts. I also include water in this category of large-block nutrients. Often overlooked, water is a vitally important component of a well-balanced diet.

Protein

Protein is made up of amino acids. Your body needs protein to build and maintain muscle, repair tissues, reproduce cells, maintain hormone function, and strengthen your immune system.

There is often confusion about identifying proteins, particularly in distinguishing between complete proteins and incomplete proteins, and learning how to combine them in a healthy, balanced diet. Complete proteins contain all of the essential amino acids. These high-quality proteins are easily digested and used by the body. Egg whites are considered the highest-quality protein—they're easy for our body to assimilate, and they are the standard used in determining protein quality. In addition to egg whites, high-quality sources of protein include fish, chicken and turkey (white meat is better for you), lean beef, low-fat cottage cheese, tofu, and whey or soy protein powder.

Incomplete, or complementary, proteins are plant proteins that lack one or more of the essential amino acids. As a result, these proteins are less efficient and/or useful for your body and should be combined with other foods to create a complete protein. For example, combining beans with rice results in a complete protein that contains all essential amino acids. There are many easy, appealing ways to combine incomplete proteins to create a serving with all the essential amino acids: Whole-wheat bread and

For Strong Bones, Get Your Vitamin D

Vitamin D is getting a lot of attention these days, and it's no wonder why: Vitamin D has been shown to cut the risk of certain cancers by 40 percent, as well as prevent osteopenia (the precursor to osteoporosis) and osteoporosis.

In a recent Harvard study of 47,000 men, it was reported that vitamin D reduced the risks of cancers of the digestive system by 43 percent. Another study from the University of California at San Diego showed a daily dose of vitamin D may reduce the risk of breast cancer by 50 percent.

What's more, vitamin D helps your body absorb more of the calcium that you consume through food. Your skin produces vitamin D when you're exposed to sunlight, but depending on where you live and what your lifestyle is like, it's tough to get enough sun to satisfy your body's need for vitamin D. Good food sources of vitamin D include seafood such as salmon, sardines, and mackerel.

The National Institutes of Health recommends that adults up to age 50 receive 200 IU (International Units) of vitamin D daily. People ages 51 to 70 need 400 IU, and people older than 70 need 600 IU.

peanut butter, whole-grain toast and a glass of milk, and whole-grain cereal with skim milk are a few examples.

RECOMMENDATIONS

- 10 to 35 percent of your total daily calories should come from protein.
- Eat a serving of protein with each meal.
- Combine your plant protein sources to create complete proteins.

Fats

Fat often gets a bad rap, but the truth is that fats are an important macronutrient in your diet. Fat provides fuel for you to burn, provides a cushion for your organs, and maintains cell membranes, and it helps your body to absorb fat-soluble vitamins, which in turn help give your skin a healthy glow. However, because fat acts as a flavor enhancer, it is all too easy to wind up with too much fat—and the wrong kind of fat—in your diet. When it comes to including fat in your daily diet, it needs to be the right fat in the right amounts.

Fat sources can be divided into three basic categories: healthy fats, fats to be used sparingly, and fats to avoid altogether. Healthy fats are unsaturated fats found in vegetable oils, nuts, seeds, and fish. The best sources of healthy fats are olive oil, canola oil, flax oil, nuts, fish oil, and avocado. Fats to be used sparingly are saturated fats found in meats and dairy. Fats to avoid are trans fats which have been linked to myriad health problems, including heart disease. Trans fat is created by a process in which hydrogen is added to vegetable oil to make it solid, so that foods can last longer. Trans fat is found in processed foods like margarine, cakes, cookies, crackers, breads, snack foods, and even "health-food" bars.

RECOMMENDATIONS

- 20 to 30 percent of your total daily calories should come from healthy fats.
- Include healthful fat in every meal.
- Use fats sparingly—a little bit goes a long way.
- Use vegetable stock, chicken stock, tomato juice, or water in place of oil to help limit your fat intake.

Carbohydrates

Carbohydrates are your body's primary fuel source. Your muscles need carbs to function, as do your brain and central nervous system. Carbohydrates break down into sugar (glucose then glycogen) in your body. When your body gets the right carbohydrates, your blood-sugar levels will stabilize, which means you will feel less hungry and maintain even energy levels throughout the day. Examples of carbohydrates include vegetables, fruits, grains, pastas, sweets, and many dairy products, like milk and yogurt.

Variety is the key to a diet balanced with healthy carbohydrate sources. There are so many choices among healthy, high-fiber, nutrient-filled carbohydrates. The best carbohydrate sources are colorful vegetables, fruits, and berries; whole grains; and low-fat or nonfat yogurt. Diets high in fiber reduce the risk of heart disease, obesity, and diabetes, as well as help reduce cholesterol.

Not all carbohydrates are alike, however. Starchy, sugar-filled carbohydrates cause your blood sugar levels to rise quickly. These foods will give you a quick boost in energy, but it's temporary, and your blood sugar levels will drop just as quickly. You'll feel that familiar "crash," mentally, physically, and emotionally. You'll start craving those same foods to lift your body from its low. Pretty soon you're in a constant cycle of crashing and craving. To avoid this exhausting, unhealthy roller coaster, stay away from starchy and sugary carbs like white bread, white rice, crackers, cookies, cakes, pies, candy, sweetened yogurts, and ice cream. Not only do these types of carbs send your blood sugar spiking,

they also have little nutritional value and are considered "empty calories."

RECOMMENDATIONS

- 45 to 65 percent of your total daily calories should come from carbohydrates.
- Eat a serving of high-fiber carbohydrate at every meal.
- Avoid sugars and starchy carbohydrates. Stay away from white foods like rice, bread, and crackers.

Water

Technically, water is not considered a macronutrient, but there is no other contribution we make to our bodies on a daily basis that is more important to our health. At nearly 70 percent, our bodies are mostly made up of water, and our blood is about 90 percent water. We can go a few weeks without food, but we can only survive a few days without water. The average person loses 2 to 3 liters of water every day, through sweat, urine, respiration, and cellular function.

And yet, so many people go through their days dehydrated. The signs of dehydration are lack of energy, confusion, headaches, body aches, irritability, moodiness, muscle cramps, and fatigue. Dark-colored urine may also be a sign of dehydration.

Sugar and Your System

The body has two primary fuel sources: fat and sugar (also called glycogen). Carbohydrates—all carbohydrates—turn into sugar in your body. This sugar becomes the fuel source glucose and then glycogen. Glucose gets converted into glycogen and is stored in your muscles and liver to be used as fuel. Once these stores are full, the excess is then rerouted—it's like a waterfall spilling over into your fat stores. It's actually the easiest way for your body to produce and store fat. This is one of the reasons why low-carbohydrate diets are so popular. When the body reduces carbohydrates to a certain level, it causes glycogen depletion and causes your body to burn primarily fat as its fuel source. Unfortunately, these days fast-burning carbs are a major part of the SAD (standard American diet), and it is this diet that is creating a generation at risk for fatty liver disease. These quickly digested foods include breads, cereals, quick oats, white rice, potatoes, and a host of other packaged foods. These are the same types of foods fed to fatten geese to make foie gras (goose liver pâté). High-glycemic diets send our blood sugar soaring, triggering a boom in insulin production by the pancreas, which in turn causes the liver to absorb the sugar (carbs) to store as fat.

The best thing we can do for ourselves is steer away from high-glycemic foods and incorporate low-glycemic, fibrous foods in their natural state, with minimal processing. Your daily diet should include fresh, nonstarchy fruits and vegetables like apples, pears, peaches, and berries. When buying "whole-grain" foods, opt for foods in their most natural state: old-fashioned oatmeal instead of instant oatmeal, brown rice instead of white rice, and whole-wheat pasta instead of regular pasta. A glycemic index list of foods is available in the Food Facts section.

Water and Your Workout

To prepare for an exercise session, drink 8 to 10 ounces of water 30 to 60 minutes beforehand. If you are working out for 60 minutes or less, you don't need to worry about drinking during your session. Just make sure you drink immediately after your workout and then throughout the day. If you are working out for more than 60 minutes, be sure to take water along with you. Bringing a small snack is also a good idea.

Thirst is a sign that your body is already moving toward the state of dehydration. Don't wait until you are thirsty to drink water. Eight cups per day is a generally recommended minimum, but with your Outdoor Fitness exercise, you may need more than that. Drinking 2 liters of water throughout the day will keep you hydrated, thinking clearly, feeling energized and satiated, and prepared for your regular fitness sessions.

Micronutrients

Micronutrients are vitamins, minerals, and trace elements found in foods. You need miniscule amounts of these nutrients to complete a healthful diet. If you're eating a well-rounded diet with a variety of colorful fruits and vegetables, you should be getting the micronutrients your body needs. For this reason I don't

prescribe supplements with the Outdoor Fitness program. A high-quality multivitamin is a good idea, however. Think of it as nutritional insurance—a way to fill in any gaps in your whole-food diet.

Your 11-Point Game Plan to Lose Fat, Retain Muscle, and Maintain Your Healthy Lifestyle

You've got all the raw materials you need to change the way you eat and incorporate food into your daily life. Now it's time to bring it all together, with a few additional tips to help you eat well for both health and pleasure. Follow these guidelines day in and day out to change your body composition, energize your system, and maintain a strong, fit, healthy body for a lifetime.

Power Foods

Power foods are super-healthful foods that provide our bodies with many benefits. Try to incorporate the following power foods in your regular eating plan:

Dark berries and blueberries. These colorful fruits are rich in fiber, vitamin C, antioxidants, and phytonutrients for good health.

Broccoli. This cruciferous vegetable is packed with nutritional power from fiber, calcium, vitamin E, vitamin C, and protective compounds like lutein and beta-carotene.

Wild salmon. The abundance of omega-3 fatty acids found in this fish reduces the risk of heart disease, stimulates the immune system, and might even reduce the incidence of depression.

Spinach. Loaded with antioxidants, vitamin C, and vitamin K, it can help you to think more clearly.

Kiwi. Did you know that this fuzzy fruit has more vitamin C than an orange? And it's loaded with fiber and potassium, too.

Garlic. Garlic has a purifying effect that reduces cholesterol, lowers blood pressure, and fights unfriendly bacteria and possibly viruses.

Tomatoes. Packed with antioxidants, vitamin C, potassium, and carotenoids, these red beauties also contain lycopene, a phytochemical proven to protect against cancers, especially prostate cancer.

Egg whites. All protein, no fat. With only six to ten calories per egg white and all the essential amino acids, egg whites are the perfect protein source.

Old-fashioned oatmeal. Perfect for endurance athletes and those in need of long-lasting energy, oatmeal is a proven cholesterol reducer and is high in soluble fiber, iron, magnesium, selenium, zinc, folic acid, and other B vitamins.

Almonds. For glowing skin and more. Rich in phytochemicals, raw almonds have been shown to decrease cholesterol and are an excellent source of vitamin E, magnesium, zinc, selenium, copper, potassium, and iron.

1. **Eat frequently.** Starting with breakfast, make sure to eat every few hours. Plan your meals and snacks for the day, a total of three main meals and two to three snacks. Eating this way will rev your metabolism and keep your system running steadily and evenly all day long.

2. **Eat whole foods.** Fresh, colorful, seasonal, and local foods are the easiest, most healthful way to keep your diet on track and provide you with the variety you need to nourish your body and mind.

3. **Eat a balance of foods.** Mix things up! Strive for an array of colors, textures, and types of food on your plate. Include protein, carbohydrates, and a small amount of healthy fat in every meal.

4. **Practice portion control.** Since you're eating many times during the day, you should be able to master the art of portion control without a problem. Remember: A palm-size serving of protein, a fist-size serving of carbohydrate, and a fingertip-size amount of fat is what you need at every meal.

5. **Cut out the fake food.** Packaged, processed foods are full of fat, salt, sugar, and chemicals. They've been stripped of their nutritional value and offer you nothing but calories and a spike in your blood sugar. Steer clear of noodle soups, salad dressings, flavored yogurts, waffles, pancakes, crackers, cereals, and cookies. Even "natural"-looking products can be loaded with junk. Spend your calories eating fresh, whole foods. You'll quickly lose your taste for the bad stuff.

6. **Become a label reader.** Always check the content of the food you purchase. Red flags include "-ose" at the end of an ingredient on a label, which indicates a type of sugar. Sucrose, dextrose, fructose, galactose, maltose: You'll often see as many as four or five of these in a single product. There's no nutritional value here—only empty calories.

7. **Drink lots of water.** Don't let yourself get thirsty. Get in the habit of drinking water throughout the day, especially before and after your workouts. When you're exercising regularly, you need about 2 liters per day. Lose the sodas and sugary drinks—you'll make a huge cut in your calorie and sugar intake if you avoid them and stick to water or decaffeinated iced tea. Use a water purifier rather than buying your water in plastic bottles.

8. **Look for the 100-calorie cut.** Find 100 calories to cut from your diet every day. What's 100 calories? A tablespoon of mayonnaise, 6 ounces of wine, a slice of bread, a chunk of cheese, a dollop of whipped cream. This is a great way to shave calories a little at a time, up to 36,000 calories per year. That's 10 pounds!

9. **Eat slowly.** A recent study has shown that people who eat slowly consume 70 fewer calories per meal. In the course of a week, that amounts to 1,500 calories! A slow, relaxed meal brings you greater satisfaction and leaves you feeling satiated while eating less.

10. **Give yourself a free meal.** Even the most dedicated, determined, and organized of us need a break. Every week or so, allow yourself one meal to eat whatever you feel like—no guilt, no recriminations. This will actually help you stay on track over the long haul.

11. **Don't eat for any reason other than hunger.** Of course it sounds obvious, but we all eat for reasons that have nothing to do with being hungry. Anxiety, boredom, and stress all send us to our cupboards. Distractions and our busy lives also lead us to eat when we're not actually hungry. How often do you eat while driving, cooking, working, reading, or watching TV? Too often, we combine eating with relaxing and socializing, and studies show that this can lead to consuming twice as many calories.

CHAPTER 10

Most Commonly Asked Questions and Answers

Whether it's a client during a one-on-one session, a caller to my radio show, or a visitor to my Web site, I field thousands of questions about health, well-being, and exercise. Here I've collected the most common and useful questions from exercisers of all skill levels. From nutrition to weight control to exercise, these questions come from people using Outdoor Fitness. What better way to end this book than in the spirit of community and conversation that Outdoor Fitness has created among thousands of people around the world?

I hope as you finish this book and continue your Outdoor Fitness journey, you will move forward with joy and confidence toward this remarkable new phase: your new fit, healthy life, lived so much more in the great outdoors.

Exercise and Lifestyle

1. Why is stretching important? Should I stretch before and after my workouts, or just after?

Well, the jury is still out, and the research is inconclusive. Some research has indicated it can decrease power in your muscles. Many people, including myself, believe in stretching major muscles after a good warm-up, but some researchers feel it could be counterproductive because your heart rate drops. I say, so what? Just build it back up again. All experts agree that we should stretch after our workouts. It's the most productive and safest time because the muscles are warm and pliable.

Here's a good rule of thumb: Warm up for 5 to 10 minutes. If anything feels particularly tight, like your hip flexors, hamstrings, quadriceps, or calves, stop and stretch them. And always stretch

Your Secret Weapon—The Golgi Tendon Organ

Muscles and their connective tissues are protected by a sensory organ known as the Golgi tendon organ (GTO), located in the junctions of muscles and their tendons. The GTO responds to increased muscle tension or contraction exerted on the tendon by inhibiting further muscle contraction. When a muscle is stretched or pulled, this natural protective mechanism signals the central nervous system and causes the muscle to relax, protecting the muscle from damage. When the tension is very extreme, its relaxing effect on the muscle can prevent an injury. You can activate your GTO by holding your initial stretch for 5 seconds, and then backing off for 5 seconds. Now resume the stretch as you normally would, holding for 20 to 30 seconds.

after your workouts. You'll prevent injuries and feel great.

Tips to remember:

- Never stretch a cold muscle. Always warm up for at least 5 to 10 minutes before stretching. On chilly days, extend this warm-up to 15 or more minutes.
- For best results, activate the Golgi tendon organ (GTO): Hold a stretch for 5 seconds, release for 5 seconds, and then execute the stretch again.
- Hold a stretch for 20 to 30 seconds, or for a total of three diaphragmatic breaths.
- Inhale to prepare for a stretch and exhale slowly while lengthening the muscle.
- Outdoors, be well aligned and evenly balanced on your terrain.

2. How can I stretch my back when I don't have a spot to lie down?

One of my favorites is the tree hang. You can also use monkey bars at your local playground. Hang from the branch or bar, take a deep breath in, and exhale slowly as you relax and release your lower back. Repeat this stretch two to three times.

> **TIP:** Lower back pain and tightness can often occur after running, especially on hard surfaces. To protect your back, run on pavement instead of sidewalks and concrete. The best surfaces for running are grass and dirt trails.

You can also use a parking meter, post, or tree. Lace your fingers just below chest height around the prop and bend over to lengthen your backside, pressing back through your hips. Manipulate the stretch by pressing into your spine and rolling up between your shoulder blades. Bend your knees and stand up.

3. What are the best exercises to lift up my rear end?

We all would like to have a toned and tight rear end. The goal here is to lift muscle. There are three main muscles in your gluteal area: gluteus maximus, gluteus medius, and gluteus minimus. To target these muscles, use these four exercises:

- Take the stairs: Go up the stairs with a full foot, pressing firmly through your heel as you step up.
- Add a kick-back by lifting your leg behind you and squeezing your glutes.
- Do my hill squats on an incline, like a grassy slope. Press through your heels as you stand up.
- Do your lunges! Lunges are great for sculpting and lifting your backside. To really target your glutes, focus on your landing and on pressing into your forward heel.

> **TIP:** Don't forget to warm up. On colder days you'll want to lengthen your warm-up from 5 to 10 minutes to about 10 to 20 minutes.

4. It's too cold where I live for Outdoor Fitness! How can I still do one of your workouts?

All right, so the weather outside may be changing from warm to cold, but don't let that interfere with your Outdoor Fitness routine. Your body is remarkably adaptive to hot and cold weather. In general, it takes 7 to 14 days to acclimate to temperature changes. The best way to adapt is to simply continue with your routine season to season. The right clothing and the right attitude will keep you on the program throughout the year.

Here's some inspiration for you: According to a study from the University of Tennessee, exercising in the fresh air on chillier days burns 12 percent more calories than the same workout performed behind closed doors—and it can burn up to 32 percent more fat, as your body has to work harder to insulate itself.

5. I live in a large city where the air pollution can get really bad. Should I be worried about breathing that dirty air?

Air quality is a concern for everyone. Exercising outdoors in some cities may put people at a greater risk for complications from frequent exposure to ozone than for those who do not. Ozone is pollution formed from the emissions of cars and trucks, wood-burning stoves, chemical or industrial plants, and refineries. These pollutants have a chemical reaction to heat and sunlight. Exposure to ozone can irritate the respiratory system and aggravate asthma.

If you believe the air quality is suspect, take precautions. The U.S. Environmental Protection Agency (EPA) has produced an Air Quality Index (AQI) to make it easy to understand the current air-quality conditions. The index has a range from zero to 500; the higher the value, the higher the level of air pollution in the atmosphere. Anything above 150 is considered unhealthy.

Find out the AQI in your city by listening to local forecasts or by logging on to the EPA Web site at www.epa.gov.

By the way, if outdoor pollution and ozone seem a little unnerving, consider the following information from the EPA:

> Indoor air levels of many pollutants may be two to five times, and occasionally, more than 100 times higher than outdoor levels. Indoor air pollutants are of particular concern because most people spend as much as 90 percent of their time indoors.

6. How can I firm and tone my legs without creating bulk?

Concentrate on doing cardiovascular workouts most days of the week: run, walk, and swim. Keep heavy-duty stair climbing to a minimum, which can add bulk to your legs. Rather than using weights, use your body's own weight to tone and shape your legs. Lunges, lateral presses, sumo squats, and leg lifts all work effectively to tone without adding bulk.

7. What is the best method to burn fat and calories: a short, high-intensity workout or a lower-intensity workout that lasts longer?

Proportionately, you'll burn more fat by exercising at a slower pace for a longer time. However, the total amount of fat and calories you burn will be lower in a less intense workout. To effectively burn fat and calories, you need to combine time and intensity to your workout routine. Remember, it takes a deficit of 3,500 calories to burn one pound of fat! Here are a few tips to incorporate greater intensity to your workouts:

- Use interval training. Run hard for 1 minute and easily for 2.
- Use hills and steps. Push your intensity up the hill and recover on the return trip down.

• Use your local track. Sprint the straightaways and jog or walk the turns.

This doesn't mean you should forsake low-intensity workouts. Far from it. Mix up your workouts throughout the week: One day is a slow-jog session, and another day is a stair-training workout.

8. I try to exercise a few days a week. Why am I not losing weight?

Losing weight isn't easy. Here are the basic steps we all must adhere to when we want to lose fat:

• *Try* is a lie. Make the decision: I will lose weight.
• Schedule your daily exercise. This means six days per week, written down on your calendar.
• Mix things up. Cardio, resistance, and flexibility training are all important components of reshaping your body composition. Add cross training into your schedule to keep your body guessing and working hard.
• Write down everything you eat and drink throughout the day. Studies show that people who do this not only lose weight, they keep it off.
• Calories count. Do not exceed 1,500 to 2,000 calories per day. It takes 3,500 calories to lose a pound of fat. A quick walk or moderate jog of 3

miles burns about 300 calories. Cut 200 calories from your diet (a glass of wine and a slice of bread), and you'll hit a 500-calorie-per-day reduction, enough for a pound a week!
• No excuses. Take responsibility for your success or failure. Own this process. Make the time. It's your life.
• Get excited! You can do this!

9. Why do my feet hurt when I get out of bed in the morning? I am getting worried it's affecting my workouts.

If your heels feel bruised and sore, you may have an overuse condition known as plantar fasciitis, which affects the thick band of tissue (or fascia) that runs under the sole of your foot, connecting your heel to the base of your toes.

Plantar fasciitis is common in runners, walkers, and people who stand for hours every day—especially in heels. Often the condition is caused by tight calves, and simple stretches take care of the problem.

If you don't treat the condition, it can become chronic and put a real damper on your exercise routine. Rest and ice is the first step in treating plantar fasciitis. Ice for 20 minutes three to four times throughout the day. An anti-inflammatory like ibuprofen will help to alleviate any pain or inflammation. Rolling a golf ball underfoot is a technique that feels good and can also regenerate tissue under the soles of your feet.

10. How do I get six-pack abs?

It's all about the right exercise and a clean diet!

First, keep this in mind: Your core is made up of two layers, the inner unit and the outer unit. The deepest layers of your core are the inner unit, made up of stability muscles. These muscles act as a natural weight belt, holding our insides in place like a girdle. The surface layers of your core are the outer unit, and these are the thick pumping muscles just under the skin.

It's important to strengthen your entire core. For flat abs and a tight waist, you must work both the inner unit and the outer unit. The fastest way to do it is to mix it up. Exercises that have you bending, squatting, lifting, twisting, and rotating will tone your torso and help you to burn the fat that lies over and between your muscles. Strengthening these muscles will also prevent lower-back pain. The TVA/ab flattener exercise in chapter 5 will tighten your inner core muscles.

Don't skip the cardio—at least 30 minutes in your aerobic zone four or more days per week. Also, eat fresh food from the earth. The fitter you get, the cleaner you'll *want* to eat. You'll naturally steer clear of the junk food aisle.

11. Should I work out when I am sick?

If your symptoms are from your neck up, ask yourself: Do I feel like working out? If the answer is yes, you're good to go. If your symptoms are located below your neck—difficulty breathing, chest tightness, wheezing, or coughing—don't exercise. Take the time to rest and recuperate.

12. How can I avoid getting bored with my workout?

The best exercise program is a simple one. Notice that I said simple, not easy! Follow these simple suggestions to sidestep workout boredom:

- Choose activities you like. The best exercise program positively stimulates the body, mind, and emotions. Fun should be of the utmost importance in your workouts.
- Remember how smart your body is. Your body will adapt quickly to exercise, and before you know it, you've reached the dreaded plateau. Don't do the same workout—like running or stair climbing—more than two days in a row. On the third day, do something different.
- Mix it up! Alternate your activities and add a new one every few months. A

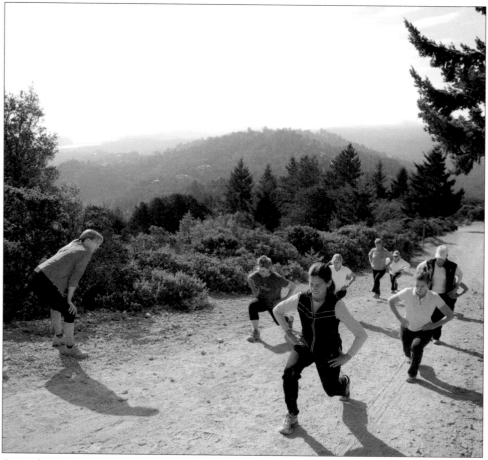

Group workouts are motivating!

few months ago, I added surfing to my routine.

• Find an exercise buddy or a workout group. It helps to have company and to be reminded that you're not alone in your struggles or your achievements. Also, you'll be sure to show up if you know someone else is counting on you.

13. How do I stay fit on the road?

On your next trip, why not sweat and sight-see at the same time? Trade in the treadmill for a self-guided running tour. Sight-jogging is a great way to get your exercise in and do a little touring at the same time; all you need is a map and a little planning. Here are a few tips to get you headed in the right direction:

- Put on your running shoes and head out first thing in the morning, before streets and sidewalks get congested.
- Many hotels have "runners' maps" that detail routes in the area. Or print out several maps of the area before you leave home and plan a new scenic loop each day.
- Wear a small, snug waist pack to hold your camera, map, and other items you'd like to have on hand.
- Avoid running through cemeteries, national monuments, and religious landmarks as it can be viewed as disrespectful.

For your safety:

- Wear light-colored clothing to make yourself visible.
- Whenever possible, use the sidewalks and walking paths.
- Stay focused: Drivers turning into an intersection will often look out for cars, but not for runners and walkers.
- Be on the lookout for unfamiliar terrain, like potholes, cracks, and crevices that can cause you to trip and fall.

14. I am way too busy to exercise. How can I fit it in?

This is the question I hear the most. Here's the thing—most people perceive lack of time as the enemy, but it's simply not true. Time management is the skill that needs to be addressed. Have you ever noticed that the busiest people get the most done? All it takes is one hour to change your entire life. Get to bed one hour earlier so that you can get up one hour earlier. The plan is to roll out of your bed and into your shoes. Set your gear out the night before.

Don't make the mistake that so many people make, thinking that they'll exercise later, at the end of the day. That's when life can get in the way, and you will feel crunched by traffic, kids, family, carpooling, and so on. I stopped training people during the after-school and after-work hours; it just became too frustrating. I only train people first thing in the morning, and rarely does anything come between my clients and their workouts.

15. You talk about the benefits of mental focus. While I understand the concept, I am unable to make progress in my own life. I find it very frustrating.

We can't solve our health and fitness issues by searching "out there"—that's because the answers are inside of you. You know what's best for you; you always have. The key to finding the answers is to get quiet, settle down, settle in, and listen to your internal voice—your heart, your soul, and, yes, your body, too. Ask yourself empowering questions: Who do I want to be? What do I want to do with my life? How do I want to move in the world? How do I want to live my life? Listen to the answers. Pay attention. Connect.

The easiest and most inspiring places to do this are in nature. Nature is your safe place, your haven, and your counselor. It is a place for Thanksuary, the core of your core—a place to connect with the natural world.

16. During the winter I feel like I don't perform as well, and I lose my motivation during my workout. What can I do to get motivated in cold weather?

Many people experience performance declines—not feeling as strong, as much endurance, or as much mental focus. It may feel like it has to do with the weather, when in fact, it may be due to dehydration. The cooling effect of air, snow, and rain can mask our sense of fluid loss—so we may fail to hydrate during a workout. Add to this the layering of clothing involved, which increases fluid loss through sweat. In fact, studies have shown a 4 to 8 percent loss of total body mass in athletes working in cold environments. What to do? Follow these three words of advice: Hydrate, hydrate, hydrate.

Don't wait until you're thirsty to drink. Drink 8 to 12 ounces before your 30- to 60-minute workout and then immediately following. To prevent dehydration, it is best to sip on fluids throughout the day until urine flows clear to pale yellow.

17. I understand the benefits of mental focus, but I am lousy at the practice. I get caught up in the "rabbit trails" you talk about.

It's called "practice" for good reason. I often tell my clients to find the right environment. Research has shown that our environment can contribute up to 70 percent in the battle of reducing stress and reducing stress hormone levels in the body, so it's important to get yourself in the right environment. Surround yourself with the calming effects of nature by paying attention to what's around you: colors, textures, the rhythm of the ocean, the crispness of the air, the scent of trees and flowers. Whether you are walking, running, lunging, or even sitting, concentrate on what is happening at that very moment—every part of it, from how you are breathing to how the air feels on your skin.

The key is to focus just on the task. This enables your brain to change through what's called neuroplasticity and take on this new practice of changing your mental focus. Start with one minute and move on from there. If you find that you begin to hop from thought to thought, come back to your breath, your posture, and your immediate surroundings.

Nutrition and Weight Control

1. Should I eat before working out or exercise on an empty stomach?

The answer is controversial at best. It all depends on your fitness goals, the intensity of your workout, and the timing. In general, you can stoke your metabolism to burn even more calories during your workout if you eat ahead of exercise. This may seem counterintuitive, but your body needs calories to burn calories. If you consistently start your workout depleted of energy, your body is inclined to hold on to its fat, entering what is often called "starvation mode."

Now having said that, if your goal is to lose fat and you go out for a 30- to 60-minute jog first thing in the morning, your body will be low on energy, or glycogen, a source of fuel your body uses while you sleep, and you can access your fat stores for fuel. I don't recommend doing this every day, however; a few times a week is fine, and you'll see results.

If your goal is athletic performance, you'll want to give your body some fuel. You might not feel hungry when you first get up, but you should eat a little something—you won't perform at your best, and you may cut your session short, if your muscles are depleted. You don't need much; 100 to 200 calories will do. Good preworkout foods include half a banana, a few pieces of dried fruit and a couple of nuts, a handful of dry cereal, or a slice of toast.

If you're working out later in the day, then it's all about the intensity of your workout. If you're simply going for a 30-minute walk, you may not need anything at all. If you are doing a more intense workout, such as weight training, interval training, a lengthy bike ride, or a long run, you'll want to give your body some complex carbohydrates to help fuel your system. Again, a 100- to 200-calorie snack is good.

2. What are the best strategies for eating healthy when eating out?

You don't have to throw your health plan aside when you go to a restaurant, but you should know that restaurant food is often loaded with fat, in the form of butter, oil, cheese, and rich sauces. Fat, after all, is a flavor enhancer. It helps to have some strategies prepared ahead of time, before you head out to eat:

- Know the menu and the venue. Check out the restaurant's menu online ahead of time and plan exactly what you'll eat. If you are headed to a party or event, find out what to expect. Often it's best to eat a little something before heading out so that you won't be tempted by the cheese and crackers.

- Instead of an entrée, order from the salad or appetizer menu. Combine a couple of appetizers or a salad and an appetizer.

- When ordering, look for these healthful food preparations: broiled, flame broiled, poached, blanched, grilled, roasted, smoked, or steamed. Ask for substitutions—these days, kitchens are used to switching out heavy, fattening sides for steamed vegetables.

- Avoid foods described with these words, which are signs of fatty, high-calorie food: breaded, tempura, crispy, Alfredo, béarnaise, beurre blanc, hollandaise, Parmigiana.

- One of the biggest threats to healthful eating out is the buffet table, where it's so easy to overdo. Choose the smallest plate and eat slowly. You'll be satisfied with less than you think, and you'll avoid making another trip to the line.

3. What beverages are good, and which ones should I avoid?

People spend so much time worrying about their food intake, they tend to forget that what we drink can make or break our healthy plan. Sodas, sweet coffee drinks, and alcohol all have calories, sugar, and fat. For example, a Starbucks 16-ounce cafe mocha with whipped cream has 360 calories, 19 grams of fat, and 32 grams of sugar. The 16-ounce nonfat white chocolate mocha without whipped cream has 310 calories, 6 grams of fat, and a whopping 52 grams of sugar! A regular 16-ounce coffee, however, has fewer than 5 calories, no sugar, and no fat. I order this and add a splash of unsweetened soy milk, which adds about 15 calories and less than a gram of fat.

Depending on the brand, one 12-ounce can of soda has between 40 and 50 grams of sugar—the equivalent of 10 to 12 teaspoons of white table sugar. Research suggests that sugary

TIP: Look out for sugar grams on food labels. You may be surprised to find out how much sugar is lurking in packaged foods. Remember this—4 grams of sugar is equal to 1 teaspoon of table sugar.

drinks are one of the leading causes of obesity in the United States.

For alcoholic beverages, moderation is considered a maximum of one drink per day—12 ounces of regular beer (150 calories), 5 ounces of wine (100 calories), or 1½ ounces of 80-proof distilled spirits (100 calories)—for women and two drinks a day for men.

The bottom line is that water is what's best for you. If you need morning caffeine, choose regular black coffee with low-fat or skim milk or unsweetened soy milk.

4. How should I cope with "snack attacks"?

Don't fight your snack attacks—just make the right choices. Nancy Clark, a nutritionist and author of the *Sports Nutrition Guidebook*, points out that "not snacking is bad practice, especially for active people." Snacking prevents cravings and keeps you from getting too hungry. Here are Nancy's key points to keep in mind about snacking:

- A snack is a snack, not a meal. Keep snacks under 300 calories.
- Choose wisely: carrots over carrot cake and apples over apple pie.
- If you're snacking before a workout, make sure you include a carbohydrate, which you'll find in unsweetened yogurt or a piece of fruit.

- Stay hydrated. Sometimes when you feel hungry, you're really thirsty.

5. What is the effect of a fatty meal on my body?

Even one fatty meal can have a negative effect on your health, by reducing the ability of your arteries to respond to the increased blood flow that occurs after such a meal. Studies have shown that blood flow is impaired for two to five hours after a fatty meal. There's some good news, though, if you can't resist chowing down on a burger and fries: A recent study shows that a brisk 45-minute walk taken within two to four hours of a high-fat meal can improve blood flow and negate potential damage to your arteries. You don't have to suit up for the gym; just get out and walk your dog, run some errands, and enjoy the fresh air.

Does this mean you can have your cake and eat it too? Not really. A healthy diet does not include foods loaded with fat and cholesterol. But because there are always occasions when we want to break the rules, you can indulge without guilt now and then—as long as you take that walk!

6. How do I avoid holiday and vacation weight gain?

The good news is that the average American gains only one pound between Thanksgiving and New Year's. The bad news is that extra pound lingers on most of our bodies all year long. Follow these five tips to avoid putting on holiday pounds:

- Keep up with your exercise appointments. Do your workouts no matter what. Include 10 extra minutes of cardio each day by walking to your errands, taking the stairs, and parking at the far end of the lot.
- Keep a food log. Experts agree you'll achieve the greatest success if you faithfully record every single thing you eat. Set a caloric goal for the day and stick with it.
- Know your weakness. If it's sweet desserts, decide ahead of time to indulge a little bit, not a lot.
- Eat before you party. Never arrive to a holiday gathering hungry or dehydrated. A 200-calorie snack, with protein and fiber, will stabilize your blood sugar and prevent binging.
- Enjoy the spirit of your vacation or holiday. These special times are about having a great time with people you love. Seek good company and enlivening experiences rather than eats and treats.

7. I need to lose some weight fast. How do I do it?

It's happened to all of us at one point or another: A special event creeps up on you, and you suddenly are anxious to drop a few pounds quickly. Here's a short-term diet and exercise plan to help you shed a few pounds fast. This is not a long-term diet plan! Use this only for a very short period of time.

- Eat mini meals (four to five per day).
- Eat lean protein with no sodium: water-packed tuna, poached chicken breasts, egg whites, whey protein powder.
- Avoid bread, pasta, rice, potatoes, and cereal.
- Avoid sugars, including fruits like bananas, grapes, and apples.
- Eat berries only in the morning.
- Eat lots of fiber-rich vegetables, such as salads and cucumbers.
- Drink at least 10 glasses of water daily.
- Exercise daily: two 30-minute cardio sessions, in the morning and the evening, plus resistance training two to three times per week.
- Two to three days before the event, cut out salt, dairy, and wheat.

8. I am trying to lose some weight by cutting out white foods like rice, bread, and pasta. I do feel a lot better mentally and physically, and I am definitely not as moody! What can I substitute instead of bread and rice?

A good substitute for pasta is a product on the market called shiratake, a Japanese noodle made of soluble plant fiber and soy. It is low in calories and carbohydrates and comes in a variety of pasta shapes.

You can use vegetables to take the place of bread and crackers. For example, use cucumber slices and red, yellow, or orange peppers in place of crackers. You can create a sandwich out of lettuce leaves instead of bread: Iceberg, butter, and red and green leaf lettuce make excellent wraps. Take one or two leaves and lay them out flat, then fill them with slices of turkey, chicken, tofu, tuna, or salmon; tomatoes; red onion; and your favorite mustard or salsa. Roll it or fold it up like a burrito.

9. Help! I've been doing a lot more business travel, and I've put on 10 pounds in two months! The problem is that I travel to different time zones, and by the time I arrive, I'd rather take a nap than exercise.

Sounds like a little preparation and planning would be helpful:

- Exercise beforehand. If you are traveling over several time zones, get some exercise in before your flight. Even a 20-minute aerobic session can do wonders to help you relax on your lengthy journey.
- Plan your workouts before you leave. Call the hotel beforehand to find out about local trails, parks, bike rentals, and sports facilities that are nearby.
- Check the weather. If you're prepared mentally and physically for inclement weather, you're more likely to follow through with your outdoor workouts.
- Pack with exercise in mind. Pack your workout stuff, including sunscreen.
- Stay with the program. You'll be more successful if you exercise at or near the same time of day you normally do—plus you'll wipe out any stress associated with falling off your routine and better adjust to the time zone change.

ACKNOWLEDGMENTS

This program began in the heights of the Sierras and made its way to the California beaches, the center of Manhattan, and nearly everywhere in between.

Hundreds of clients, students, trainers, friends, and colleagues have participated in its evolution and have enthusiastically provided feedback that continues to improve it.

For the implementation and realization of this book, I extend my deep gratitude to:

John Coghlan for your unwavering love and support in all my endeavors.

My family for your understanding of my need to "hang from trees."

Kearney and Callan Coghlan for occasionally hanging from trees with me.

My clients for your continued excitement to be part of the Outdoor Fitness movement; I will always remember our adventures on the trails.

Susan Gonzalez, my first client and dear friend, who long ago envisioned the "Outdoor Fitness movement."

Harvard biologist E. O. Wilson, who coined the term biophilia. Your work has helped many of us understand why we feel at home outdoors.

Dr. Howard Frumkin for your invaluable work and your explanation of how and why nature is the most valuable contributor to our health.

Dr. Candace Pert for your concept of BodyMind, a continuous source of inspiration to me.

Warren Witherell, who showed me how to start and stay focused on this work. The shoebox got full!

Dr. Adrian Rawlinson and California Pacific Orthopedic and Sports Medicine for your support, input, and implementation of the successful Outdoor Fitness Body Composition Study.

John Abdo for your generosity and enthusiasm in helping me to shape the Outdoor Fitness Body Composition nutritional program.

My literary agent Debra Goldstein, who gets it done!

Billie Fitzpatrick, my collaborator, for positivity, creativity, and "getting it."

FalconGuides editor, Scott Adams, for your enthusiasm and vision, and Julie Marsh for invaluable editing and production assistance.

Marisa Klein and Geoff Vaughan for your generosity and time to pose for photos!

Special thanks to Mother Nature and her power to heal, inspire, provide, and energize.

FOOD FACTS FOR MAXIMUM FITNESS AND OPTIMAL WEIGHT

You Need to Eat!

Your resting energy expenditure, or Basal Metabolic Rate (BMR), is how many calories your body needs just to function on a daily basis. This number does not include activities other than normal bodily functions like the beating of your heart, the functioning of your internal organs, and the blinking of your eyes. A realistic weight loss is one to two pounds per week. Any more than that is not considered sustainable or particularly healthy.

While you're not required to count calories, keep in mind for fat loss to occur, it will be important that you consume a reduced number of overall calories. You'll get very good at eating the right foods, in the right amounts and at he right time.

- Women: No fewer than 1,200 calories per day
- Men: No fewer than 1,500 calories per day.

A Word about Portions
Start "Eyeballing" Portions

As you are creating a routine and learning the caloric content of the foods you eat, I'd like you to also understand portion sizes.

Portion Control

When you understand what constitutes a portion, you won't have to count calories ever. I believe part of the reason that more than 65 percent of Americans are overweight is due to the fact that portion sizes have ballooned to "super-size."

What is a Portion?

Protein is about the size of a deck of cards or the palm of your hand (the palm—not fingers, too!).

Carbohydrate is about the size of your fist. Think a small apple.

For chopped fruits, vegetables and cooked whole grains, a portion is about what you can hold in your cupped hand (½ cup).

For cereal and berries, it's about the size of a baseball (1 cup).

> **TIP:** Become familiar with the caloric content and correct serving size of what you eat and record it.
> - How many calories are in the foods you eat?
> - What is the correct portion size?
> - Write it down—know what you've put in your body.

Fats and oils should be used sparingly. One tablespoon is 14 grams of fat and approximately 100 calories.

Peanut butter is about the size of a walnut (2 tablespoons).

For hard fats, like butter and cheese, think of a pat of butter or the tip of your index finger.

Meal Planning: Feeling Satiated and Satisfied

Food Combining

To feel satisfied, think clearly, and keep your energy up and even, you will want to combine a portion of protein with a portion of carbohydrate, and a little fat, at each meal.

Choose nutrient dense foods—the more variety, the better. Draw from the list below and mix it up. Eat seasonally—for color, flavor, and nutrients.

How Often Should I Eat?

Five to six times a day: three main meals and two to three small meals.

Why?

Eating early and often creates a metabolic reaction in your body—and stokes and strengthens the engine.

Ever notice when you don't eat breakfast, you aren't hungry until noon or later? However, after that initial meal, you become ravenous and may even end up binging.

When you eat breakfast, you start the engine, and when you continue to gently feed the engine, you'll burn fuel more efficiently, and you'll burn more body fat.

Eat every few hours and you will maintain and gain lean muscle mass, burn excess fat, and lose the cravings, because you'll maintain even blood-sugar levels, lose the hunger, and have more energy. You'll even think more clearly and be less grouchy!

Bottom Line

Losing fat and maintaining your ideal body composition is not about deprivation. It is about creating healthy habits that you can maintain and incorporate into your lifestyle.

For best results, choose a "cut-off" time, a time in the evening to end all eating, two to three hours before going to bed. Don't worry if you feel a little hungry. That's your body telling you it's burning calories! After a week or so, you'll get into the routine and feel fine with it. You may enjoy creating a new evening routine—settling into a cup of flavorful decaffeinated tea, for example.

Losing Fat Is Not about Deprivation

It is about creating healthy habits that you can maintain and incorporate into your lifestyle.

Burn, Baby, Burn!

The body has two primary fuel sources: fat and sugar (glycogen). Let me explain what is meant by "sugar." Carbohydrates, all carbohydrates, turn into a sugar in your body. This sugar becomes the fuel source glucose and then glycogen. Glycogen is stored in your muscles and liver, and once these stores are full, they're full! The excess is then rerouted into your fat stores. It's actually the *easiest way* for your body to produce and store fat. This is one of the reasons why low-carbohydrate diets are so popular: When the body reduces carbohydrates to a certain level, it causes glycogen depletion and prompts your body to burn primarily fat as its fuel source.

What Should I Eat?

Fresh, colorful, seasonal foods are loaded with nutrients and will fill you up. Make sure that at each meal you include a portion of protein (about the size of a deck of cards) and a portion of carbohydrates from the columns below. Be sure to include an extra serving of vegetables in at least two of your daily meals (see Meal Templates).

The Good Stuff, a Sample Food List

Fibrous Carbohydrates

Artichokes (steamed or boiled)

Asparagus

Broccoli

Brussels sprouts

Cabbage

Cauliflower

Celery

Collard greens

Cucumbers

Eggplant

Green beans

Lettuces

Mushrooms

Onions

Peppers (green, red, yellow)

Snow peas

Spinach

Sprouts

Tomatoes

Turnips

Yellow squash

Zucchini

Simple Carbohydrates

Blueberries

Blackberries

Cantaloupe

Cherries

Grapefruit

Kiwi

Lemons

Limes

Milk (nonfat)

Oranges

Peaches

Pears

Plums

Raspberries

Strawberries

Yogurt (plain, nonfat)

Complex Carbohydrates

Multigrain hot cereal

Old-fashioned oats

Whole-grain cereal

Vegetables and Legumes

Beans

Red potato (small)

Sweet potato (small)

Breads and Crackers

Bran-a-crisps

Pita (whole-grain)

Ryvita (multigrain)

Sprouted Wheat

Whole Grains

Barley

Bulgur

Brown or wild rice (½ cup cooked)

Quinoa

Protein

Beef tenderloin

Buffalo

Chicken breast (no skin)

Cornish hens (no skin)

Deli meats (low-fat, low-sodium)

Lean ground beef

Lean ground turkey

Lean ham

Pork tenderloin

Top round

Top sirloin steak

Turkey breast (no skin)

Veal chop

Veal top round

Abalone (no breading)

Calamari (no breading)

Cod

Crab

Haddock

Halibut

Lobster

Mackerel

Oysters, mussels, and clams

Prawns

Salmon (fresh and canned)

Scallops

Sea bass

Shrimp

Snapper

Tuna (fresh and water-packed canned)

Protein, Dairy

Cheese (fat-free or low-fat [1–2% fat] varieties)

Cottage cheese

Egg whites and egg substitutes

Tofu (low-fat or light variety)

Unsweetened soy milk

Protein Powders

Egg white

Unsweetened soy

Unsweetened whey

Fatty Proteins (Use sparingly!)

Almonds

Brazil nuts

Cashews

Peanut butter, (1 teaspoon)

Peanuts

Pistachios

Walnuts

Feta cheese

Mozzarella

Parmesan

Provolone

Ricotta

String cheese

Oils (1 tablespoon =100 kcal=14 fat grams)

Flax oil

Olive oil

Peanut oil

Soybean oil

Walnut oil

Fat Alternatives

Chicken stock

Tomato juice and water

Vegetable stock

Herbs, Spices, and Sweeteners

Extracts

Herbs (all fresh and dry)

Lemon and lime juice

Spices without sugar

Spike™

Stevia™

Xylitol™

Condiments

Capers

Horseradish

Hot sauce

Ketchup, unsweetened

Mustards (no sugar)

Pepper (all varieties)

Pickles (except sweet)

Salsa (no sugar)

Soy sauce (low-sodium)

Tamari

Vinegars (wine and cider)

Beverages

Water!

Club soda with a splash of fruit juice

Coffee and tea

Decaffeinated herbal teas

Mineral water

Mineral water with lemon or lime

Unsweetened iced teas

What Will It Take to Lose Unwanted Pounds?

Unfortunately, when it comes to losing fat, exercise alone is simply not enough. To lose one pound of fat, you must burn through 3,500 calories. With my program you're not required to count calories; however, it is important that you understand the caloric density (content) of the foods you eat, as well as what constitutes a serving size. One of the most helpful things you can do (especially in the beginning) to lose unwanted pounds and gain muscle is to record what you eat and how often you eat it.

Take a pass on:

Most processed and packaged foods
    Refined carbohydrates
    Refined sugars
    White flours and "processed whole wheat"
    Remember:
• Sugars come in many forms.
• Sugars are calorically dense carbohydrates with no nutritional value.
• During digestion all carbohydrates (except the fiber) are broken down into the sugars glucose and glycogen.

Foods High in Sugar

Asian chili sauce (check sugar content)
BBQ sauce
Candy
Cocktail sauce
Condiments
Ice cream
Jams and jellies
Ketchup
Power bars, energy bars
Sugar and sugar-laden foods

Beverages

Colas and sodas
Fruit juices
Liqueurs and cordials
Smoothies
Sports drinks, Gatorade, etc.

Starchy Carbohydrates

Breads and bagels, white and wheat
Cakes
Cereals
Cookies
Donuts
Matzoh
Pasta
Pastries
Pretzels and crackers
Quick oats and packaged oatmeal
Rice and rice products, rice cakes
Rolls
Pies
White flour

Dairy

Cream

Cream cheese

Frozen yogurt

Fruit yogurts (all)

Full-fat cheeses

Half and half

Ice cream

Milk (full-fat)

Sour cream

Fats

All trans fats

Butter (use sparingly)

Margarine

Fructose

Fruit juice concentrate

Glucose (dextrose)

High-fructose corn syrup

Honey

Inverted sugar

Lactose

Maltose

Molasses

Raw sugar

Rice syrup

Sugar

Table sugar (sucrose)

Check the Label for Hidden Sugars:

Brown sugar

Cane sugar

Corn sweetener

Corn syrup

TIP: A food product is likely to be high in sugar if one of the above terms appears as one of the top-three ingredients or if several of the terms are listed.

What about Alcohol?

Alcohol contains sugar! Consume in moderation . . .

What counts as a drink?

12 ounces of regular beer

5 ounces of wine

1.5 ounces of 80-proof distilled spirits (100 calories)

GLYCEMIC INDEX LIST OF FOODS

HIGH GLYCEMIC INDEX FOODS (ABOVE 85)*

Angel food cake
Bagel (white)
Bread (barley flour)
Bread (white)
Cheerios
Corn bread
Corn chips
Cornflakes
Couscous
Croissant
Cream of Wheat
Dates

Doughnut
English muffins (plain)
Grape-Nuts
Honey
Ice cream
Maltose
Molasses
Maple syrup
Muffins
Pancakes
Potato
Potato chips

Pretzels
Raisins
Rice cakes
Rice Krispies
Rye flour
Saltine crackers
Sodas
Sports drinks
Special K Cereal
Sucrose
Waffles

MODERATE GLYCEMIC INDEX FOODS (60-85)

Banana
Bulgur
Bread (oat bran)
Bread (7-grain)
Bread (whole wheat)
Buckwheat
Cake (sponge)
Cereal (oat bran)

Corn (sweet)
Grapes
Grapefruit juice
Ice cream (low-fat)
Kiwi
Mango
Oatmeal (quick cooking)
Orange juice

Pita (white)
PowerBar
Rice (basmati)
Rice (brown)
Rice (white)
Sweet potato
Tortilla (corn)

LOW GLYCEMIC FOODS (BELOW 60)

Apples (whole)
Apricots
Barley
Beans
Berries (all types)
Bread (9-grain)

Chickpeas
Grapefruit
Hummus
Lentils
Nuts
Oranges

Peaches
Pears
Plums
Rice Bran
Soup (tomato)
Soup (vegetable)

*White bread used as the reference food (GI = 100)

MEAL TEMPLATES

As you begin to integrate your workouts into your daily routine, you can maximize your fitness and lose weight, if that is one of your goals, by keeping track of your meals. Use this meal template to record your food choices. Soon this exercise will be second nature. But for the first few weeks, remember to write down your meals.

B = Beverage

Carb-C = Complex Carbs

Carb-F = Fibrous carbs

Carb-S = Simple carbs

Pro = Protein

Day 1 Date _____

Meal 1 (6–8 a.m.)

Carb-S _____

Carb-S _____

Pro _____

B _____

Meal 2 (2–3 hours after previous)

Carb-S _____

Pro _____

B _____

Meal 3 (2–3 hours later)

Pro _____

Carb-F _____

Carb-F _____

B _____

Meal 4 (2–3 hours later)

Carb-C _____

Carb-F _____

Pro _____

B _____

Meal 5 (6–7 p.m.)

Pro _____

Carb-C _____

Carb-F _____

B _____

Meal 6 (9 p.m. or 2–3 hours before bed)

Pro _____

Carb-F_____

Total Calories_____

Exercise_____

Day 2 Date _____

Meal 1 (6–8 a.m.)

Carb-F _____

Carb-C _____

Pro _____

B _____

Meal 2 (2–3 hours after previous)

Carb-Si _____

Pro _____

B _____

Meal 3 (2–3 hours later)

Pro _____

Carb-F _____

Carb-F _____

B _____

Meal 4 (2–3 hours later)

Carb-C _____

Carb-F _____

Pro _____

B _____

Meal 5 (6–7 p.m.)

Pro _____

Carb-C _____

Carb-F _____

B _____

Meal 6 (9 p.m. or 2–3 hours before bed)

Pro _____

Carb-F _____

Total Calories_____

Exercise_____

Day 3 Date_____

Meal 1 (6–8 a.m.)

Carb-C _____

Carb-S _____

Pro _____

B _____

Meal 2 (2–3 hours after previous)

Carb-S _____

Pro _____

B _____

Meal 3 (2–3 hours later)

Pro _____

Carb-F _____

Carb-F _____

B _____

Meal 4 (2–3 hours later)

Carb-C _____

Carb-F _____

Pro _____

B _____

Meal 5 (6–7 p.m.)

Pro _____

Carb-F _____

Carb-F _____

B _____

Meal 6 (9 p.m. or 2–3 hours before bed)

Pro _____

Carb-F_____

Total Calories_____

Exercise_____

Day 4 Date_____

Meal 1 (6–8 a.m.)

Carb-S_____

Carb-S _____

Pro _____

B _____

Meal 2 (2–3 hours after previous)

Carb-S _____

Pro _____

B _____

Meal 3 (2–3 hours later)

Pro _____

Carb-F _____

Carb-F _____

B _____

Meal 4 (2–3 hours later)

Carb-C _____

Carb-F _____

Pro _____

B _____

Meal 5 (6–7 p.m.)

Pro _____

Carb-C _____

Carb-F _____

B _____

Meal 6 (9 p.m. or 2–3 hours
before bed)

Pro _____

Carb-F_____

Total Calories_____

Exercise_____

Day 5 Date_____

Meal 1 (6–8 a.m.)
Carb-F _____
Carb-C _____
Pro _____
B _____

Meal 2 (2–3 hours after previous)
Carb-S _____
Pro _____
B _____

Meal 3 (2–3 hours later)
Pro _____
Carb-F _____
Carb-F_____
B _____

Meal 4 (2–3 hours later)
Carb-C _____
Carb-F _____
Pro _____
B _____

Meal 5 (6–7 p.m.)
Pro _____
Carb-C _____
Carb-F _____
B _____

Meal 6 (9 p.m. or 2–3 hours
before bed)
Pro _____
Carb-F _____

Total Calories_____
Exercise_____

Day 6 Date_____

Meal 1 (6–8 a.m.)
Carb-C _____
Carb-S _____
Pro _____
B _____

Meal 2 (2–3 hours after previous)
Carb-S _____
Pro _____
B _____

Meal 3 (2–3 hours later)
Pro _____
Carb-F _____
Carb-F _____
B _____

Meal 4 (2–3 hours later)
Carb-C _____
Carb-F _____
Pro _____
B _____

Meal 5 (6–7 p.m.)
Pro _____
Carb-C _____
Carb-F _____
B _____

Meal 6 (9 p.m. or 2–3 hours before bed)
Pro _____
Carb-F _____

Total Calories_____
Exercise_____

Day 7 Date_____

Meal 1 (6–8 a.m.)

Carb-S _____

Carb-S _____

Pro _____

B _____

Meal 2 (2–3 hours after previous)

Carb-S _____

Pro _____

B _____

Meal 3 (2–3 hours later)

Pro _____

Carb-F _____

Carb-F _____

B _____

Meal 4 (2–3 hours later)

Carb-C _____

Carb-F _____

Pro _____

B _____

Meal 5 (6–7 p.m.)

ANYTHING GOES MEAL!

B _____

Total Calories_____

Exercise_____

RESOURCES

Abdo, John. *Foolproof Eating Plan*. New York: St. Martin's Gifford, 2002.

———. *Make Your Body a Fat Burning Machine*. New York: St. Martin's Gifford, 2002.

Agatston, Arthur. *The South Beach Diet: The Delicious, Doctor-Designed, Foolproof Plan for Fast and Healthy Weight Loss*. New York: St. Martin's Press, 2005.

American College of Sports Medicine, American Dietetic Association and Dieticians of Canada. "Nutrition and Athletic Performance" 2000: 2130–2141.

Apter, M. J. "Reversal Theory and Personality: A Review." *Journal of Research in Personality* 18 (1984): 265–288.

Baerg, W. J. "The black widow and five other venomous spiders in the United States." *Arkansas Agr.* 408 (1959): 1–43.

Baker, Beth. "Happy by Nature." *Washington Post*, June 4, 2002: HE01.

Barbour, AG. *Lyme Disease: The Cause, the Cure, the Controversy*. Baltimore: Johns Hopkins University Press, 1996.

Ben-Shahar, Tal. *Happier*. New York: McGraw-Hill, 2007.

Billings, J. "An Overview of Task Complexity." *Motor Skills: Theory into Practice* 4 (1980): 18–23.

Bryant, Cedric X., and Daniel J. Green, eds. ACE *Personal Trainer Manual: The Ultimate Resource for Fitness Professionals*. San Diego: American Council on Exercise, 2003.

Burton, L. M. "A Critical Analysis and Review of the Research on Outward Bound and Related Programs." Unpublished doctoral dissertation, Rutgers University, New Brunswick, NJ, 1981.

Bush, S. P. "*Spider Envenomations, Widow*." eMedicine Journal. Jan 2002. www.emedicine.com/EMERG/topic546.htm.

Carter, Albert E. *The New Miracles of Rebound Exercise*. Nature Distributors, 1988.

Chek, Paul. *How to Eat, Move and Be Healthy!* San Diego: Self published, 2004.

Clark, Linda. *Rejuvenation*. Greenwich, Conn.: The Devin-Adair Co., 1979.

Cohen, Michael J. *Reconnecting with Nature: Finding Wellness through Restoring your Bond with the Earth*. Minneapolis: Ecopress, 2007.

Comtech Research. "What are ions?" www.comtech-psc.com.

Cox, R. H. *Sport Psychology: Concepts and Applications*, 4th ed. pp. 112–120. Boston: McGraw-Hill, 1998.

Davis-Berman, J., and D. S. Berman. "Early Wilderness Programs" (ch. 3) in Wilderness Therapy: Foundations, Theory & Research. Dubuque, Ia.: Kendall/Hunt Publishing, 1994.

De Geus, J. C., J. P. Van Doornen, and J. F. Orbebeke. "Regular Exercise and Aerobic Fitness in Relation to Psychological Make-up and Physiological Stress Reactivity." Psychosomatic Medicine 55 (1993): 347–363.

Driver, B., R. Nash, and G. Haas. "Wilderness benefits: a state of knowledge review." Proceedings: national wilderness research conference: issues, state-of-knowledge, future directions. R. C. Lucas, compiler, 1987.

Duffee, R. A., and R. H. Koontz. "Behavioral effects of ionized air on rats." Psychophysiology 1965 Apr 1(4): 347–359.

Durstine, J. Larry, ed. ACSM's Resource Manual for Guidelines for Exercise Testing and Prescription, 2nd ed. Philadephia: Lea & Febiger, 1993–2003.

Foss, M. L., and S. J. Keteyian. Fox's Physiological Basis for Exercise and Sport pp. 267–539. New York: McGraw-Hill, 1998.

Foster, Robin. "Sights and Sounds of Nature Ease Pain: Soothing therapy helps patients during lung procedure." HealthScoutNews, May 24, 2004.

Frumkin, Howard. "Beyond Toxicity: Human Health and the Natural Environment." American Journal of Preventative Medicine, April 2001.

Gen. Tech. Rep. INT-220. Ogden, Utah: U.S. Dept. of Agriculture, Forest Service, Intermountain Research Station, pp. 294–319.

Giannini, A. J., B. T. Jones, and R. H. Loiselle. "Reversibility of serotonin irritation syndrome with atmospheric anions." J Clin Psychiatry March 1986, 47 (3): 141–143.

Goodwin, Sarah. "Frumkin's Rx: Intense exposure to natural elements." Emory Report. April 9, 2001. www.emory.edu/EMORY_REPORT/erarchive/2001/April/erApril.9/4_9_01frumkin.html.

Hendler, Sheldon Saul. The Oxygen Breakthrough. New York: Simon & Schuster, 1990.

Hooker, Richard. "Arete." 1996. www.wsu.edu/~dee/GLOSSARY/ARETE.htm.

Howard, Pierce J. The Owner's Manual for the Brain—Everyday Applications from Mind-Brain Research. Austin: Bard Press, 2006.

Ilg, Steve. The Winter Athlete. Boulder, Colo.: Johnson Books, 1999.

Kaplan, R., and S. Kaplan. The Experience of Nature: A Psychological Perspective. Cambridge, England: Cambridge University Press, 1989.

Kripke, Dan F., Sonia Ancoli-Israel, Jeffrey A. Elliott, and Harry Klemfuss. "Light Treatment and Biological Rhythms: An Indexed Bibliography," 1st ed. (March 1993)

Kuo, Frances, and William Sullivan. "Coping with Poverty: Impacts of Environment and Attention in the Inner City." *Environment and Behavior,* January 2001: 33(1):5–34.

Lemonick, Michael D. "The Power of Mood." *Time* Magazine. Jan. 12, 2003:161(3).

Loehr, James E. *The New Toughness Training for Sports.* New York: Plume, 1994.

Louv, Richard. *Last Child in the Woods—Saving Our Children from Nature Deficit Disorder.* Chapel Hill: Algonquin Books, 2006.

Luttgens, Katherine, and Nancy Hamilton. *Kinesiology—Scientific Basis of Human Motion.* New York: McGraw-Hill, 1997: 297–309.

Mann, Denise. "Negative Ions Create Positive Vibes." www.WebMD.com.

Mitchell, B. W., and D. J. King. "Effect of negative air ionization on airborne transmission of Newcastle disease virus." *Avian Dis* 1994 Oct–Dec: 38(4): 725–732.

Moses, J., A. Steptoe, A. Mathews, and S. Edwards. "The Effects of Exercise Training on Mental Well-being in the Normal Population: A Controlled Trial." *Journal of Psychosomatic Research.* 1989 Jul: 33(1): 47–61.

Nedley, Neil. *Proof Positive: How to Reliably Combat Disease and Achieve Optimal Health through Nutrition and Lifestyle.* Ardmore, Okla.: Nedley, 1999: 500–501.

Neher, J. O., and J. Q. Koenig. "Health effects of outdoor air pollution." *American Family Physician.* May 1994.

Nusnick, David, and Mark Pierce. *Conditioning for Outdoor Fitness.* Seattle: The Mountaineers, 1999.

Ott, John N. *Health and Light: The Effects of Natural and Artificial Light on Man and Other Living Things.* Ariel Press, 2000.

Peper, Erik, Ph.D. *Creating Wholeness—Integrating Mind/Body/Spirit.* Institute for Holistic Healing, San Francisco State University, 1998.

Phillips, Bill. *Body for Life.* New York: HarperCollins, 1999.

Pretty, Jules, Murry Griffin, Martin Sellens, and Chris Pretty. "*Green Exercise: Complementary Roles of Nature, Exercise and Diet in Physical and Emotional Well-Being and Implications for Public Health Policy.*" CES Occasional Paper, University of Essex. March 2003.

Rossman, B., and Z. J. Ulehla. "Psychological Reward Values Associated with Wilderness Use: A Bifunctional-Reinforcement Approach." *Environment and Behavior,* 1977, 9(1):41–65.

Schloss, P., and D. C. Williams. "The serotonin transporter: a primary target for antidepressant drugs." *Journal of Psychopharmacology* 1998, 12(2): 115–121

Schwarzenegger, Arnold. *The New Encyclopedia of Modern Body-building.* New York: Simon & Schuster, 2007.

Sears, Barry. *The Top 100 Zone Foods: The Zone Food Science Ranking System.* New York: Harper, 2004.

Shaw, Johnathan. "The Deadliest Sin: From Survival of the Fittest to staying fit just to survive: scientists probe the benefits of exercise—and the dangers of sloth." *Harvard Magazine.* 2004: 34–43.

Shields, Jack. "The Central Propulsion of Human Thoracic Duct Lymph" (film). Santa Barbara, Calif. 1980.

Solderitsch, C., and R. Meyer. "*Is Our Modernizing Culture Killing Biophilia?*" Ohio State University Study Paper, 2000.

Taylor, J., and G. S. Wilson. "Intensity Regulation and Sport Performance" in J. Van Raalte and B. Brewer, eds. *Exploring Sport and Exercise Psychology* 2nd ed., 99–130). Washington, D.C.: American Psychological Association, 2002.

Thayer, R. E. *The Origin of Everyday Moods: Managing Energy, Tension, and Stress.* New York: Oxford University Press, 1996.

Thoms, Lesley. "Back to Our Roots for Serenity?: Ecopsychology in Improving Well-Being." *The Psychologist,* July 2003, 16(7): 356–359.

Ulrich, R. S. "View through a Window May Influence Recovery from Surgery." *Science,* 1984, 224: 420–421.

Wansink, Brian. *Mindless Eating: Why We Eat More Than We Think.* Bantam Books, 2006.

Wilson, Edward O. *Biophilia,* Cambridge, Mass.: Harvard University Press, 1984.

Young, Lisa R. *The Portion Teller: Smartsize Your Way to Permanent Weight Loss.* New York: Broadway Books, 2005.

Young, R., and R. Crandall. "Wilderness use and self-actualization." *Journal of Leisure Research,* 1984, 16(2): 149–160.

Zilber, Steven A. "Review of Health Effects of Indoor Lighting." *Architronic,* 1993: 2(3).

WEB

American Academy of Dermatology: www.aad.org

American Medical Association: www.ama-assn.org

The site of the International Community for Ecopsychology lists recommended readings, counselors, and upcoming events: www.ecopsychology.org

www.johnvdavis.com/ep/benefits.htm

National Institutes of Health: www.nih.org

Taylor, Jim. Seminar handouts and Web site: www.alpinetaylor.com

INDEX

E AUTHOR

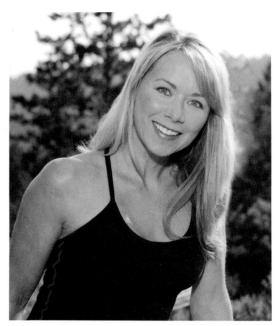

MITCHEL SHENKER

...te fitness insider,
...oor Fitness, the
...program in the
...erican Coun-
...accredited outdoor
...ior. Vindum not only travels
...country teaching her techniques to
health and fitness professionals, but as
a member of the ACE faculty, she also
gives frequent lectures at international
fitness conferences about the scientifically proven benefits of being outdoors.

Vindum hosts the weekly radio show
"Outdoor Fitness," which airs nation-
wide on the SportsByline USA Broadcast
Network and worldwide on the American Forces Radio network, on which she has
interviewed people like Joe Montana, Chris Carmichael (longtime coach to Lance
Armstrong), Governor Mike Huckabee, Dr. Mehmet Oz (author of the *You! The Owner's Manual* series), and Dr. Barry Sears (author of *The Zone*). A regular trainer
of the trainers at Nike World Headquarters, she's a featured podcaster on LIME.
com, alongside heavyweights like Neal Donald Walsch (author of *Conversations
with God*) and Dr. Andrew Weil. She's a former world champion mountain biker and
professional skier, and she wrote and starred in Gaiam's "Walking Pole."

Vindum and her programs have been featured in local, regional, and national
print and broadcast outlets, including *Self, Fitness, Prevention, Sports Illustrated for
Women, Backpacker, San Francisco Chronicle, Real Simple, Vogue, Elle, Los Angeles
Times, New York Times,* and countless others. The proud owner of several Falcon-
Guides, she lives in San Francisco, California.